BUTTE
AND THE 1918
INFLUENZA
PANDEMIC

BUTTE
AND THE 1918
INFLUENZA
PANDEMIC

JANELLE M. OLBERDING

THE
History
PRESS

Published by The History Press
Charleston, SC
www.historypress.com

Cover images courtesy of Butte–Silver Bow Public Archives.

First published 2019

Manufactured in the United States

ISBN 9781467143264

Library of Congress Control Number: 2019932639

COMMUNICATION IN THE COPPER mines of Butte, Montana, in the early twentieth century happened through a system of bells and whistles. The bell system helped underground miners communicate with those on the surface, while the whistles allowed the mines to send messages to the entire city. Mostly, the whistles signaled the beginning and end of shift. They also blew when something was wrong—when there was a cave-in or fire or when men were trapped underground. The whistle of the affected mine blew first, and the others would then pick up and copy its signal to notify the entire city.

WHEN THERE WAS A major disaster, the whistle of each mine in Butte blew shrilly ten times.

CONTENTS

CONTENTS

ACKNOWLEDGEMENTS

This book was a labor of love. Though I'd like to say it was always a joy, that's simply not the truth. The research, calculating, mapping, charting, writing, and revising took hours of hard work, some sweat, and even a few tears. The end result is the culmination of a lifelong dream, and I am so grateful for those who poured their own time into this project.

My biggest debt of gratitude is to my family. My husband, Mark, has heard more about influenza in the last few years than he probably ever thought possible. He read, reread, commented, and discussed the manuscript at length; put up with all my trips to and talk about Butte; and drove over four hundred miles across Montana on Christmas Day so that I could spend part of our family vacation doing research. I'm immensely grateful to him and our daughter for their patience and support through the long days and nights of graduate school and the years that followed as I took this project so much further than originally intended. Thank you for always believing in me, loving me, and supporting me through this journey. I know it wasn't always easy.

Dad, Mom, and my sisters were my first supporters. Thank you for always believing in me and, believe it or not, "letting" me proofread your work. The joke's on you—all the editing made me a better writer.

Much appreciation goes to Ron Jackson, a talented and successful writer and historian in his own right. Thank you, Ron, for your extensive read-throughs, all your thoughtful comments and suggestions, and your willingness to spend hours on the phone, answering all of my questions and sharing your knowledge of writing, editing, and publishing. Thanks most of all for your support and encouragement. You made a difficult journey so much easier.

My friend Jamie Broaddus went above and beyond editing this manuscript for me. Thank you, Jamie, not only for your time and work on editing the complete manuscript but also for answering all of my random texts asking about grammar, punctuation, phrasing, and word choice. I owe you books, coffee, cat paraphernalia, and good conversation for years to come.

Thanks also go to Lynn Newnam for volunteering as an early reader, providing suggestions and never hesitating to share and discuss the latest news on all things related to communicable disease. Few others can match my level of interest and enthusiasm regarding potentially deadly communicable health threats.

Thank you to the staff of the Montana Historical Society in Helena for safeguarding our state's rich history and helping me navigate through all of your resources.

This book truly would not be possible without the Butte–Silver Bow Public Archives and its dedicated and helpful staff. Director Ellen Crain and her staff gave a tremendous amount of help, support, and suggestions as I attempted to wade through the treasure-trove of documents and resources they care for. A special thank-you goes to Nikole, Aubrey, and Kim for their help in obtaining resources and photos. Thanks also go to the Archives for allowing me to speak on this topic in their facility on more than one occasion. Whenever you are in Butte, make sure to stop in to their beautiful building and thank the Archives staff for all their hard work in guarding and sharing Butte's incredible history.

Thanks also go to the Butte Historical Society and Cim LeProwse for inviting me to speak on this topic in Butte. It was an honor and a pleasure to visit with you all, and your enthusiasm for an early version of this work helped me believe that I might have an audience for the book.

Butte's World Museum of Mining and Mai Wah Society are just two of the amazing places to visit and conduct hands-on research in Butte. I highly recommend adding them to your list of places to see when you visit.

Finally, thank you to the caring and dedicated public health professionals of yesterday, today, and tomorrow. I'm privileged to have counted myself among your ranks.

WRITER'S NOTE

This is a work of nonfiction.

In March 1918, my grandfather Benjamin Scheffelmaier was born in Elgin, North Dakota. He was the youngest of four and the only child born in the United States to my great-grandparents Christof and Karolina, immigrants from what is now Ukraine. Christof, according to family history, was a very strong, compassionate, and helpful person. He helped his neighbors when influenza struck their small farming community until he contracted influenza as well. Christof died on November 20, 1918. He was thirty.

This piece of family history lodged in my mind years ago, and when I began a career in public health, I started learning more about influenza and other communicable diseases. I also learned about their often overlooked, but immensely impactful, presence in history. Over five years ago, as a graduate student, I started to study one of those important yet seemingly forgotten episodes in history—the one that killed my great-grandfather. Throughout the course of research for my master's capstone on the influenza pandemic of 1918 in Montana, my relationship with Butte began.

Butte caught my attention first through statistics. Between September 1918 and February 1919, the City of Butte filed 707 death certificates that list influenza as either the primary cause of death or a contributing factor. According to those numbers, Butte's mortality rate during the influenza pandemic of 1918–19 was two times higher than Montana's as a whole. I had to find out why.

Both the City of Butte and Silver Bow County kept death records for the city during the influenza pandemic of 1918. There is some overlap between these records. I focused my research on the deaths filed by the City of Butte, as they include only the deceased who lived within the city's boundaries. These 707 deaths are most certainly not Butte's total influenza mortalities. For reasons analyzed and discussed within this book, several deaths most likely went unreported or were listed with a different cause. However, 707 is the most accurate recorded number available and is a sample large enough to be considered statistically significant for comparison to the whole population.

In 1918, Butte was an incredibly diverse city, and failing to consider this renders any exploration of its past incomplete. When looking at influenza victims' specific demographic factors—age, gender, ethnicity, and occupation—the numbers may not add up to 707. This is because not all death certificates listed each of these identifiers. However, each individually cited factor is listed enough times to keep figures statistically significant.

Records from the 1910 census were used to calculate ratios of influenza deaths to total population in different demographic categories. Though the census was conducted eight years prior to the pandemic, it is the most complete collection of contemporary demographic information available. The population of Butte grew in the years between 1910 and 1918, and the demographic makeup undoubtedly changed, but the census numbers still provide the best and most accurate means of calculating mortality rates within the city.

The dates and actions of government officials described in this work are all true, as are the names of all individuals. No direct quotations have been attributed to people unless it is documented that they spoke those exact words.

How victims of the 1918–19 strain of influenza experienced their illnesses and deaths naturally can't be known exactly in each case. When a person's illness and/or death is described, the writer and the reader must use both fact and imagination to consider how the victim and those close to him or her actually felt. Perhaps a victim's last moments did not happen exactly as I've explained in some cases, but I hope that I have remained close enough to the specifics of the disease that I've painted a picture that could be exactly true.

What we must remember, writer and reader alike, is that the people mentioned within these pages were all real. They lived, worked, played, loved, experienced joy and sorrows, and had families and friends who cared for them. In that respect, they were not all that different from you or me. It is my sincere hope that by attempting to tell their stories—even the suffering—we can honor their memories.

Over the course of the last five years, I've spent countless hours reading public health records, devouring book after book of Butte history, collecting and recording information from death certificates, calculating statistics, exploring huge archival books of immigration and naturalization records, carefully thumbing through newspapers a century old, painstakingly marking each influenza victim's address on a huge map of Butte, and hypothesizing the reasons for Butte's suffering. I explored Uptown Butte many times, imagining cobblestone, busy shops, and streetcar bells. I walked back and forth along the Copperway Trail from Montana Tech to the yard of the Mountain Consolidated. Under the headframes, now still and quiet, I pictured men waiting to go underground and wondered how far they would be able to see through the smelting smoke to the valley below. I tried to make myself hear the constant sounds of industry and piercing mine whistles over the various hours of the day. I did all this to answer a question—to understand why Butte had suffered such a high mortality rate in 1918. In doing so, though, something else happened. As I learned, first in pages and then in person, so many of the things that made Butte so unique and so unforgettable, I discovered her heart. And then she took a piece of mine.

This is a work of nonfiction, yes, but it's also a love letter. I fell in love with Butte through her history and stories—stories that showcase her big heart and indomitable spirit. I am honored to tell one.

PROLOGUE

A pestilence isn't a thing made to man's measure; therefore we tell ourselves that pestilence is a mere bogy of the mind, a bad dream that will pass away. But it doesn't always pass away and, from one bad dream to another, it is men who pass away.
—*Albert Camus,* The Plague

Influenza is a familiar foe. Most people can tell you, roughly, when flu season occurs. We know how it feels to contract the flu, and we have heard about the ways it can be prevented—handwashing, staying away from sick people, seasonal vaccination. But if we don't take those measures, and even sometimes when we do, we may get sick. Most of us will resign ourselves to missing school or work for a few days and then recovering and moving on with life. Like taxes or road construction, influenza has become something that we are used to hearing about and dealing with at a certain time of year. We have become, to an extent, complacent.

What we forget is that the object of our complacency can kill. According to the Centers for Disease Control and Prevention, "Influenza has resulted in between 9.2 million and 35.6 million illnesses, between 140,000 and 710,000 hospitalizations, and 12,000 and 56,000 deaths annually since 2010."[1] Most of us have probably had a personal experience with influenza and come out the other side fine, so instead of worrying ourselves about influenza, we direct our worry toward the killer diseases we hear about in the news, like Ebola. While it is a deadly cause for concern, the majority of us in the United States will never have contact with Ebola. However, too often we focus on the exotic threats like that and forget about influenza—a common pathogen responsible for the deaths of thousands of Americans each year. We forget that it's a threat or at least forget to take that threat seriously.

Unlike media favorites like Ebola, SARS, and Zika, which are considered newly emerging diseases, influenza is old. The word *influenza* itself was first used in the fourteenth century to describe how the stars allegedly "influenced" disease. Influenza caused outbreaks and epidemics, possibly even pandemics, for centuries before the first recorded flu pandemic took place in 1580.[2] The disease's spread was documented across Asia, Africa, and Europe, and it likely reached the Americas, as well. Two more pandemics followed in the eighteenth century, and the nineteenth century experienced at least four.

Perhaps, then, by the twentieth century, the world was caught up in the complacency cycle that many of us find ourselves in today regarding influenza. People had lived through outbreaks, epidemics, and even pandemics. Maybe they or a family member would get sick once every year or so with the seasonal variety of the disease. Like our concerns about newly emerging diseases, our early twentieth-century counterparts probably felt that diseases like tuberculosis, typhoid, and cholera were far more worrisome.

The year 1918 began changing the way science, medicine, and individuals felt about influenza. In less than a year, the disease killed 30 to 50 million people worldwide and approximately 675,000 Americans, which is a far cry from the Centers for Disease Control and Prevention's current calculated average, even at the extreme high end. Historians estimate that approximately one-quarter of Americans suffered from the disease, with infection rates much higher in some parts of the country. The 1918–19 influenza strain was twenty-five times more lethal than average strains. It killed 2.5 percent of those infected, whereas average influenza strains kill one-tenth of 1 percent of infected individuals. For perspective, if a pandemic with the same mortality rate hit in the present day, it would kill 1.5 million Americans—more than the number that die of heart disease, cancers, strokes, chronic pulmonary disease, AIDS, and Alzheimer's combined.[3]

With the exception of Antarctica, no continent or country, province or state was spared. In the United States, Montana fared much worse than many other states. Only three—Pennsylvania, Maryland, and Colorado—suffered higher influenza mortality rates. Between August 1918 and February 1919, the disease swept across Montana's eastern plains as quickly and violently as its winds, wandered through its western forests, and climbed up and down its mountains. No community, no matter how rural or isolated, escaped. The disease infected and killed homesteaders on the prairie; timbermen in mill towns and lumber camps; cattlemen following their herds along riverbanks and streambeds; and men, women, and children who lived, worked, and played in small towns and cities statewide. Montana physicians reported over 37,560 cases of influenza, and approximately 5,000 Montanans—one out of every hundred—died of the disease.[4] The city of Butte suffered worst of all. Despite holding about 10 percent of the state's population, Butte's residents accounted for almost 20 percent of the state's influenza deaths. In fewer than six months, the disease killed approximately 1,000 people living in or around the city.[5] In the last months of 1918 and into 1919, influenza was cause for almost anything but complacency on the "Richest Hill on Earth."

PART I

BIOLOGY, LIFE, DEATH, AND THE "RICHEST HILL ON EARTH"

⌐◇◇◇⌐

What remains is Butte, America, a unique and storied city with a core group of people who still retain much of the camaraderie of the unforgiving days of underground hard rock mining, when a man's partner was his lifeline. "How's she go, Pard?" "She's gotta go!" And Butte is still going.

—*Larry Hoffman, "The Mining History of Butte and Anaconda"*

Chapter 1

THE RICHEST HILL ON EARTH

*It is a place where immigrants from around the globe planted their roots to become
Americans…A place where living one day at a time was more than just a motto,
it was a fact of life…A place where a hard day's work was demanded and a fair
day's wage was expected….Where neighborhoods met ethnic pride….This place
called Butte, Montana, is bound to leave a lasting impression on you.*
—*Pat Kearney*, Butte Voices: Mining, Neighborhoods, People

A t the western foot of the Continental Divide in southwestern Montana, a creek curves gently around the base of a hill that is taller and steeper than it looks from a distance. The creek's waters gleam in the afternoon sunlight, looking like a river of silver, the metal the hill's first settlers tried to scrape from the nearby rocks. For centuries, Native Americans used elk horns to scrape gleaming chunks of it from the dirt and rock. In the 1860s, white prospectors took up residence in search of an even more precious metal: gold. But it wasn't gold or silver that turned Big Butte, the knobby hill above Silver Bow Creek, into the "Richest Hill on Earth." It was copper.

Finding gold on and in Big Butte was rare, and though "tantalizing assays of silver" had been discovered, the ground under what would become the city of Butte, Montana, was a proverbial gold mine of copper. By the 1880s, the tentative settlement of miners' canvas tents, rough lumber shacks, and rickety lean-tos had turned into a robust town, drawing even more miners, plus entrepreneurs, would-be capitalists, and tycoons who hoped the miners would make them rich. Led by the intelligent, industrious, and often cutthroat "Copper Kings"—staunch Irishman Marcus Daly, politician and entrepreneur William A. Clark, and young upstart F. Augustus Heinze—the copper business in Butte exploded. In 1882, nine million pounds of copper were pulled out of the ground in Butte. A year later, production increased by 250 percent. By 1896, the area was producing 26 percent of the world's copper supply. Gold and silver, just byproducts of the more profitable copper mining operation, were worth $500 million a year.[6]

Such extravagant wealth created opportunity and diversity. By the dawn of the First World War, Butte's population had exploded. She was one of the largest cities in the American Rockies and the biggest in Montana by far. The 1910 census counted 39,165 people in Butte, almost three times as many as in Great Falls, the state's second-largest city. By 1918, the population had grown even more, thanks to the wartime demand for copper. One out of every 10 Montanans lived in Butte. The city offered seemingly endless opportunity for both emigrants and immigrants, the miners who came to dig copper out of the earth and those who followed to cater to their needs: their families, salesmen of all kinds, restaurateurs and brewers, tailors and seamstresses, grocers, launderers and housekeepers, financiers, railroad men, and prostitutes.

The settlement of Butte began on the hill, gradually spreading down across Silver Bow Creek and leveling along the valley floor. Her heart, though, was Uptown. Butte's downtown area was laid out in square blocks along Big Butte's face, looking across the wide valley to mountain peaks on every side. Shops, businesses, government offices, and neighborhoods of all types spread across Uptown Butte, headframes and mine yards occasionally breaking up the grid of streets.

Due to its wealth of copper, Butte was electrified early. It boasted everything other contemporary cities could offer. Street lamps glowed and streetcar rails wound through Butte, delivering members of both the working and upper class to their various destinations—mine yards, fine department stores, banks, or favorite saloons. Almost any Uptown streetcar stop was a quick walk through the cobblestoned streets to all types of businesses. Residents had a number of retail choices. They might choose to visit one of the five floors of Hennessey's, an Uptown department store, for all their needs in one place. Shoppers could find fine china, cast-iron pots, clothing, groceries, and books and stop for a drink at the soda fountain. Along the way, they might deposit or withdraw funds from their accounts within the Metals Bank Building or stop at one of Butte's over two hundred saloons. After their errands, shoppers could stop for a meal at one of the city's many

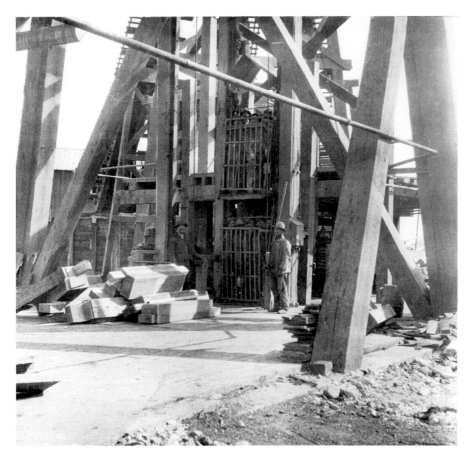

Each mine shaft had a lift system similar to that shown here. As many as ten to twelve miners would crowd into each cage for ascent and descent. *Montana Historical Society.*

restaurants—"traditional" cafés, Chinese noodle parlors, Italian bistros, or one of the many other ethnic eateries scattered about Butte.[7]

The streetcars also ran all the way to Columbia Gardens at the base of the foothills on the east end of town. Columbia Gardens, Montana's first and only amusement park, was a gift to the city from William A. Clark, and visitors could ride the carousel and roller coaster, bet on horse races, enjoy the arcade, or stroll through the park's greenhouse or around the lake. Amateur and minor-league baseball teams played here during the summer months, and dances were held in the ballroom year-round.

Columbia Gardens wasn't the only choice for entertainment in Butte. Residents could take in plays, including Broadway shows, silent movies

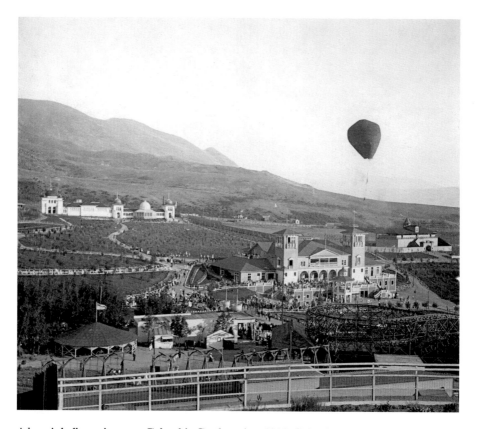

A hot air balloon rises over Columbia Gardens circa 1906. Columbia Gardens boasted a roller coaster, horse races, gardens, an arcade, baseball games, and more. *Montana Historical Society.*

and musical acts, at one of the city's many theaters. Working-class residents enjoyed watching amateur boxing matches, often held in the back rooms of Uptown saloons. Chinatown and the Red Light District offered a different type of entertainment. Residents from each stratum of Butte society might visit one of Chinatown's opium dens or one of the District's brothels, perhaps in the same night. Levels of discretion were based on the client's place in Butte's social circles and the amount he or she was able to pay. Butte offered everything that any American city could in terms of amenities, services, and vices. All of these factors helped to establish her as one of the early twentieth century's most populous and cosmopolitan cities in the northern Rockies, all thanks to copper mining.

Neighborhoods of varied wealth spread across the hillside and down to the valley floor. Men lived in boardinghouses, sharing a room and sometimes even a bed with a man who worked the opposite shift. One man rose from bed as another returned from work to take his turn in the same spot. Others lived in crowded one-room shacks, sleeping on any open floor space they could find. Entire families, sometimes of multiple generations, lived in two- or three-room houses in more classically residential neighborhoods. People lived in apartments above the shops they owned or frequented, they rented living space from families with an extra room, they moved from hotel room to hotel room on a weekly or monthly basis. They lived wherever there was space, and space was in short supply. Approximately one thousand people lived in each square block of Uptown Butte, which itself sat atop hundreds of miles of underground tunnels.

Butte was crowded but modern and full of opportunity. It was full of noise—the constant sounds of industry, mine whistles, and the voices of thousands of people   and it was dirty. Soot covered every surface, and the sky was nearly always gray and polluted from the smoke of the smelter fires that constantly burned to separate copper from rock.

The city's residents, rich and poor, came from all over the world—each part of the United States, Canada, East Asia, Central and South America, and every country in Europe. By the time copper production reached its peak in 1916, the mines printed and posted safety messages in no fewer than sixteen languages.[8] The city's neighborhoods were often delineated by ethnicity as clearly as any nation's boundary on a map.

Early twentieth-century Butte's most prestigious blocks neighbored its Uptown business district. Mine owners, bankers, and the city's most successful merchants—some of the richest men in America at the time— built large, exquisitely detailed mansions on the West Side of Uptown Butte. William A. Clark's great Butte mansion, constructed with materials from around the world and featuring every modern amenity imaginable, still sits on the West Side at the corner of Granite and Idaho Streets. The West Side was a diverse neighborhood, though. Simpler one- and two-story homes were located on the same or next block as their more impressive neighbors.

Centerville sat north of Uptown in the middle of the mining district. Since it was home to two groups of people who traditionally disliked one another— the Cornish and Irish—ethnic pride was always on display in Centerville. Each group had its own groceries, barbers, drugstores, and dry goods shops. The homes were simple and built quickly, often right next to mine yards. Little thought went into planning for infrastructure in Centerville, and the dirt-packed neighborhood lacked plumbing all the way into the 1950s.[9]

Just to the east of the Uptown business district sat Finntown, a narrow strip popular with Finnish immigrants. Most of the area's residents were single men, and Finntown's most distinguishing feature was its large number of boardinghouses. The Broadway Dining Room boardinghouse, run by Mrs. Riipi, served six hundred meals a day. Finnish miners with families who lived in other parts of town often brought their families to Finntown boardinghouses like Mrs. Riipi's for occasional meals and social visits.[10]

Finntown was bordered by Corktown and Dublin Gulch on the north and the Cabbage Patch on the south. All three were primarily Irish neighborhoods. Like Centerville, most of these neighborhoods' residents were miners and their family members. In Corktown in particular, "a number of the families were run by the mother because the father had been killed in the mines."[11] Corktown and Dublin Gulch were Butte's first neighborhoods, and most of their buildings were constructed of wood. Fires were, unfortunately, common and devastating occurrences in both neighborhoods. The Cabbage Patch, split from the other two Irish neighborhoods by Finntown and part of the business district, was much poorer than its two counterparts. The neighborhood was full of run-down shacks and shanties built of wooden grocery boxes and whatever other materials residents could salvage, sometimes from other dwellings in the area. "You tried to avoid walking through the Cabbage Patch if you could," said a former resident. "It could really smell bad there because residents threw raw sewage out into the streets."[12]

Italian Meaderville sat east at the foot of the mountains. Meaderville was one of the most polluted neighborhoods in an extremely dirty city. The area housed a number of mine dumps and smelters that sent sulfur spiraling into the air at all hours of the day. Many of Meaderville's residents spoke only Italian at home, and the neighborhood was famous for the Italian grappo served in its bars and restaurants. "I recall old women walking back from mass in the morning with their long coats and a little flask of grappo tucked away under their coats," recalled a former resident. People came to Meaderville from all over Butte for the gambling, restaurants, and bars.[13]

Chinatown and the Red Light District sat right next to each other in the heart of Uptown Butte. Chinatown was almost like a city of its own. "Residents retained the dress…of their homeland with braided queues, baggy trousers, and blouses of silk or cotton."[14] Their place of worship and meetinghouse, the joss house, was a two-story pagoda-like structure "covered with elaborate embellishments."[15] The Chinese ran laundries, dry goods stores, and noodle parlors and sold vegetables and poultry in China

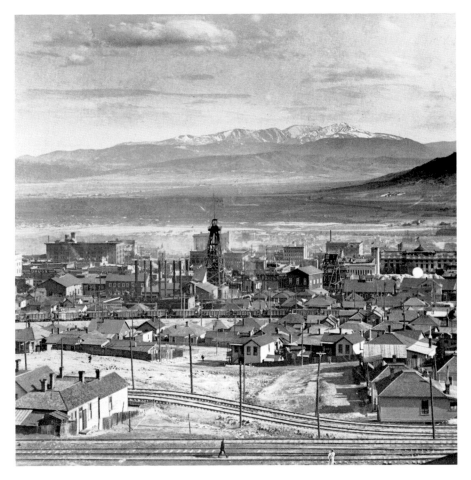

A view looking south from the Walkerville area to Uptown Butte and the mountains across the valley. *Montana Historical Society.*

Alley. More action in Chinatown happened in the tunnels below its streets. The tunnels, which connected a number of buildings along Chinatown's main street, housed illegal gambling parlors and opium dens. The Red Light District's madams and "girls" lived next to Chinatown and were frequent customers of the Chinese shopkeepers, restaurateurs, doctors, and opium peddlers. The district boasted a number of fine brothels, each run by a wealthy madam. Some women—the most beautiful and popular who could make the most money—lived in the brothels with the madams, giving the bosses a share of their earnings to keep their place in the house. Most of the district's women, though, lived in the neighborhood's back alleys in tiny, cold tin and board lean-tos. All of the district's women, especially those who made their living in Butte's dirty alleyways, lived harsh, rough, and often tragically short lives.

Central Butte ran from the southern borders of Chinatown and the Red Light District to the railroad tracks, where Butte's rich hill gradually met the flat valley floor. It was one of the city's most diverse neighborhoods, home to residents of Welsh, Irish, Scandinavian, African, Eastern European, and Mexican descent. The neighborhood held churches of various denominations and became home to Butte High School. Since it was settled later than neighborhoods higher on the hill, Central Butte's residents were less crowded than their neighbors to the north.[16]

Butte's incredible racial and ethnic diversity led to tensions as the United States entered into World War I. Germans and Serbians were afraid of how they would be treated by their French, English, and American counterparts. The ever-present Irish-English feud reached a fever pitch with Irish suspicion over English alignment with the Americans. The first United States draft registration for World War I on June 5, 1917, led to riots in Butte's streets. But once underground, the battles above ground were subject to cease-fire. The war machine needed copper, Butte needed to supply it, and each man needed to return home at the end of his shift. In the depths of the mines, each man, regardless of his language, country of origin, or political belief, knew his life depended on communicating with and trusting the man next to him. In Butte, tragedy or the ever-present threat of it was stronger than any dispute.

Even in the best of times, though, the conditions underground were dangerous and challenging. The work was hard and deadly. Miners worked ten-to-twelve-hour shifts, hundreds to thousands of feet underground the entire time. Once a man went underground, only accident, illness, or injury was cause to bring him back up before the end of shift. Accidental injury and death were, unfortunately, common occurrences. An explosion at the Granite Mountain Mine killed fifteen in 1915. A fire at the Pennsylvania in 1916 killed twenty-one. Many smaller accidents occurred each week, injuring or killing one or two miners at a time.

The worst hard rock mining disaster in American history took place in Butte in June 1917. A fire broke out in the Granite Mountain, trapping hundreds of the men working in its shaft and crosscuts and those of the neighboring Speculator Mine underground. Rescue operations lasted days. As smoke continuously poured from the Granite Mountain shaft, men made valiant attempts to pull their comrades from underground tunnels filled with poisonous gas. Time was of the essence. Men raced through the darkness to the lifts, frantically ringing the signal bell for the surface. Others began climbing from level to level on wooden ladders only to be turned back by smoke and foul, dangerous air. Dozens perished, choking, and vomiting on poison gas.

Two separate groups of miners, led by the quick-thinking and courageous Manus Dugan and J.D. Moore, quickly constructed bulkheads at dead ends of short tunnels. The bulkheads, made of scraps of wood, canvas, mud, the men's clothing, and anything else they could find, kept Dugan's group of twenty-nine and Moore's of eight alive for more than thirty-six hours after the fire started. After so many hours, though, the limited oxygen supply behind the bulkheads began to run out. After lying hungry, thirsty, mostly naked, tired, and afraid in the stifling heat for over a day and a half, they were now suffocating in their own expelled breath.

Rescuers equipped with enormous helmets and oxygen tanks eventually found Moore's group before all of their breathable air had run out. Dugan's men, though, were forced to create their own escape. After continuously and carefully testing the mine's air quality through a hole he kept plugged with a rag, Dugan eventually came to the conclusion that the air outside the bulkhead was no more deadly than the carbon dioxide–heavy air within. He instructed his men to tear down the bulkhead and race as quickly as their weakened bodies could move through the dissipating gas to safety. Ultimately, 31 of the men behind the bulkheads made it to the surface alive. Dugan and Moore were not among the survivors. Both seemed to know they would not make it. "If the worst comes I myself have no fears but welcome death with open arms," Dugan wrote to his wife in a note found later in his pocket. Moore wrote notes to his wife in his time book. "I got some boys with me in a drift and put in a bulkhead," he wrote. "You will know your Jim died like a man and his last thought was for his wife that I love better than anyone on earth." All told, 168 men lost their lives in the Granite Mountain–Speculator Disaster. Manus Dugan and J.D. Moore have, deservedly, achieved folk hero status in Butte.[17]

The disaster threw another spark on the nearly continuous flames of labor union battles in Butte. The North Butte Mining Company, owner of both the Granite Mountain and the Speculator, had a reputation for being a fair and safe company, preferable to working for the rival Anaconda Company, which owned most of the hill's holdings. A tragedy of this extent, in one of the city's "safest" mines no less, called for immediate action. Due to the long hours and dangerous conditions, labor reform had always been on the hearts and minds of Butte's miners. For decades, Butte had been a bastion for workers' unions—the Richest Hill on Earth was also called the "Gibraltar of Unionism." The battles over workers' rights spilled into Butte's streets, sometimes violent and bloody. Even deadly. After the Granite Mountain–Speculator Disaster, the struggle became even more desperate. One of its culminating moments came less than two months after the tragedy. Frank Little, an organizer for the Industrial Workers of the World, a labor union with antiwar and suspected Communist leanings, was found dead in Butte on August 1, 1917. He'd been abducted from his boardinghouse, beaten, dragged behind a car through the streets, and hanged from a railroad trestle at the edge of town. His killers left a note that included the symbol of the Montana vigilantes—the numbers 3-7-77—pinned to Little's body but were never identified. Instead of turning on one another even more, though, Butte's citizens united. Little's funeral was the largest ever in Butte history.

Butte must have felt that if she had made it through the tragic and tumultuous events of 1917, she could make it through anything. She had survived crowding, pollution, political violence, and man-made disaster. But it was another threat—tiny and natural, deadly and unstoppable—that would present one of her biggest challenges.

Butte was an exceptional city. She was socially, culturally, and economically diverse. She offered a variety of opportunities to a wide assortment of people. In the fall and winter of 1918, though, the things that made her so exceptional also helped make her incredibly cruel.

Chapter 2

MORTARS AND MICROBES

If in some smothering dreams you too could pace
Behind the wagon that we flung him in,
And watch the white eyes writhing in his face,
His hanging face, like a devil's sick of sin;
If you could hear, at every jolt, the blood
Come gargling from the froth-corrupted lungs,
Obscene as cancer, bitter as the cud
Of vile, incurable sores on innocent tongues,—
My friend, you would not tell with such high zest
To children ardent for some desperate glory,
The old Lie: Dulce et decorum est
Pro patria mori.
—*Wilfred Owen, from "Dulce Et Decorum Est"*

In the first weeks of 1918, a doctor in rural Haskell County, Kansas, found himself overwhelmed with patients, most with very similar complaints. Headaches, body aches, fatigue, fever, dry cough—these in themselves weren't uncommon symptoms. The doctor diagnosed these cases as influenza—also not uncommon—but this influenza was different. It was sudden, violent, and extraordinarily deadly, killing three of its thirteen victims. Within weeks, though, there were no more cases to report. The dead were buried, the ill recovered, and it was business as usual in Haskell County.[18]

In March, the Ford Motor Company in Dearborn, Michigan, sent approximately one thousand workers home sick with influenza, and in April and May, over one-quarter of the prison population at San Quentin in Northern California suffered from influenza. Today, influenza is a reportable disease. Local health jurisdictions are required by law to report diagnosed cases to their state health departments. An account of Haskell County's experience is available only due to one doctor's painstaking record keeping. In the early twentieth century, only formal institutions and organizations, like the Ford Motor Company and San Quentin, kept close records of non-reportable diseases. Whether other communities, businesses, and agencies had similar scenarios is hard to know for sure, but the U.S. Army's experience that spring makes it highly probable.

In 1918, the army was the largest organizational complex in the United States. Just as Haskell County was recovering, across Kansas at Camp Funston, hundreds of soldiers reported sick in March and April. Over two hundred then developed pneumonia. Though forty-eight died, this was not an exceedingly unheard-of mortality rate for pneumonia in 1918, so Funston officials took little notice. The epidemic waned after a couple of weeks, and Camp Funston concentrated once again on the business of war.[19]

But Kansas wasn't alone. From Camp Oglethorpe in Georgia to Camp Lewis in Washington State, influenza and pneumonia raged through army posts across the United States. The disease struck quickly, slowed the camps' regular operations for a short time, and then disappeared again. Many soldiers fell ill, but for the most part, only a few died. The disruption wasn't enough to stop the great war machine. Disease was unfortunately common during wartime. In each previous war, more soldiers died of disease than of wounds, and the army's modest public health force focused on illnesses it saw as bigger threats—diseases like typhus, measles, and gastrointestinal illnesses.

Despite the lack of attention the army gave it at the time, it is apparent to modern historians that the military establishment played a large role in spreading influenza in early 1918. In March, thirty-six members of the Fifteenth U.S. Cavalry were struck with influenza on the voyage to Europe. Six died. Cases of the disease appeared in Bordeaux, France, a major U.S. disembarkation point, in April. That same month, the British Expeditionary Force and French forces reported cases of influenza, and it crossed No Man's Land to the German army as well. Forces on each side had thousands of ill soldiers, and Erich von Ludendorff, head of the German army in France,

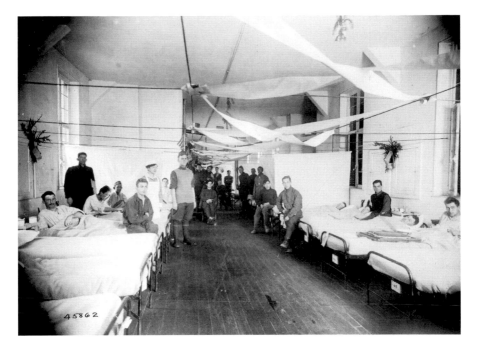

A U.S. Army influenza hospital in France in December 1918. *National Archives.*

blamed influenza for his failed July offensive. The disease spread out of the camps into nearby civilian populations. By June, influenza was prevalent in England and Wales, and by July, the disease had appeared in northern Europe, North Africa, India, China, New Zealand, and the Philippines.[20]

Though its first recorded appearance was in Haskell County, modern researchers are still hesitant to definitively pinpoint Kansas as the pandemic's origin point. Its appearance, almost simultaneously, at different points around the world was baffling. Perhaps it started in East Asia, where the proximity between human and animal reservoirs leads to more frequent development of pandemic influenza strains. Maybe it emerged somewhere in Africa, whose lands, especially its jungles, are host to a wide variety of dangerous, infectious microbes. It may have started in Europe as a simple flu outbreak but spread rapidly due to European troop movements, mutating and becoming deadlier as it went. Or maybe the answer lies in some combination of those factors.

Other contemporary theories about where the disease had come from were as varied as the names it took. The Spanish blamed the pestilence on the war-polluted air that blew over from France. Citizens of Allied nations worried

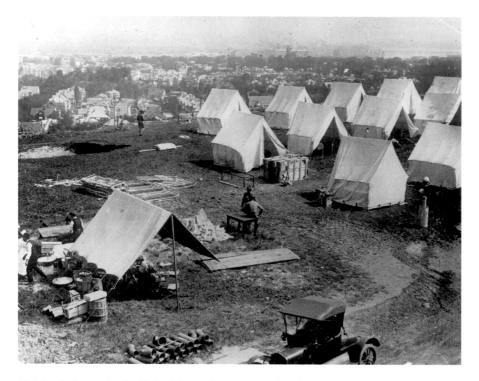

Fighting influenza in the United States Army. To combat the epidemic of influenza that had struck a number of soldiers and sailors, a special camp was fitted up on the grounds of the Correy Hill Hospital at Brookline, Massachusetts. This shows a general view of the new hospital camp. *National Archives.*

it was part of a German plot—a form of biological warfare designed to not only win the war but conquer the world. German soldiers on the Western Front called it *Blitzkatarrh*, the French *la grippe*.[21] In most places, and even into the present, it was known as "Spanish influenza," leading many to believe, falsely, that the disease originated in Spain. Spain, neutral in World War I, was simply one of the only nations to publicly discuss the pandemic, and it was international news when the country's king, Alfonso XIII, came down with the disease. The United States and other western nations hesitated to publish news of the pandemic, afraid that it would dampen support for the war effort. Officials believed publicizing the reality of the pandemic might cause worry, even panic, and hurt morale. The war, it seems, cannot be entirely separated from influenza, or influenza from the war.

If the reports of influenza in the United States early in 1918 went largely unnoticed outside of army camps and the civilian populations immediately surrounding them, it was impossible to ignore them when the disease returned with a vengeance in the early autumn. After making its way around the globe, influenza settled once again into America beginning in late August and early September. Once it returned, it ravaged each corner of the nation—army camps and densely populated cities, the frozen tundra of the Alaskan wilderness, and communities of all sizes and makeup in between. Where it had appeared before, it appeared again, but this time much more virulent and exponentially more deadly. The virus, it seems, had mutated.

Chapter 3

SHIFT, DRIFT, AND MUTATE

Although remarkable advances have been made in science and medicine during the past century, we are constantly reminded that we live in a universe of microbes—viruses, bacteria, protozoa, and fungi that are forever changing and adapting themselves to the human host and the defenses that humans create.
—"National Strategy for Pandemic Influenza," November 2005

Not all strains of influenza are created equal. Influenza types A and B are the cause of seasonal influenza cases and outbreaks each year. While both can lead to serious illness and, in some cases, death, influenza A viruses are responsible for causing pandemics. This is because influenza A viruses are instilled with a dangerous proclivity to shift and mutate over time—to change their genetic makeup—in small ways or in large ones. Sometimes the change happens over a long period, but often it occurs very quickly. This unpredictability can make influenza A viruses exceedingly difficult to prevent or treat. By the time a vaccine has been created and a population has developed some immunity to the strain, it has changed. It has adapted to all the weapons—man-made and natural—that could have been its downfall.[22]

If people were able to see the influenza virus, they may compare it to a ball with spikes or rods protruding from its surface. These are proteins: hemagglutinin (H) and neuraminidase (N). Strains of influenza A are named after what subtypes of hemagglutinin and neuraminidase they contain—H1 through H18 and N1 through N11. For example, after the "swine flu"

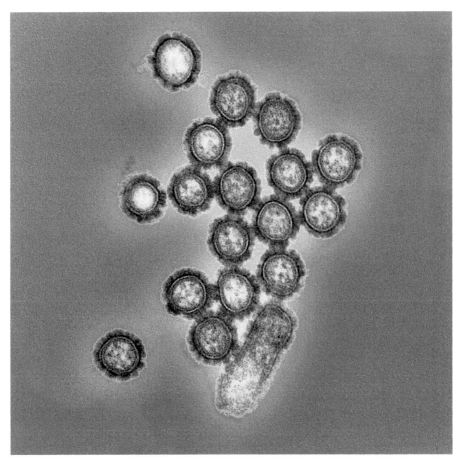

H1N1 influenza virus particles seen under a transmission electron microscope. *National Institute of Allergy and Infectious Diseases.*

pandemic of 2009, H1N1 became a household name.[23] The other influenza A that commonly circulates among humans is H3N2.[24]

Of course, that leaves 196 other possible influenza A combinations. These strains occur naturally in animals, usually pigs and birds, but also in other mammals, like bats, horses, and dogs. Avian influenza—"bird flu"—often circulates widely in poultry populations, sometimes without causing problems. In other instances, it can lead to widespread, deadly illnesses in the birds, triggering, in worst-case scenarios, mass kill protocols designed to wipe out entire flocks to prevent the spread of infection. Normally, avian influenza viruses don't affect people, but human infection with an avian virus is possible. Human infection is most common when people are in regular close contact with birds and don't wear proper protective equipment. Most human infections have taken place in the poultry farms or open marketplaces in East Asia. Avian influenza doesn't always cause a serious illness in humans. Still, it is fortunate that human-to-human transmission of avian influenza is exceedingly rare and the spread relatively limited when it has occurred. Avian influenza can be deadly. H5N1 and H7N9 strains are the avian viruses responsible for having caused the highest morbidity and mortality rates among humans.[25]

Influenza viruses found in pigs more readily infect humans than avian viruses. When detected in humans, viruses that normally infect swine are called "variant influenza viruses." Variant viruses are the wild card of influenza viruses, and swine are the ultimate reservoir. Pigs are vulnerable to swine influenza viruses and those that infect humans and birds. A backyard pig can be infected with influenza viruses from multiple species all at once. If this happens, the viruses' genes can blend themselves within the pig's body, like different chemicals being swished together in a test tube. The outcome is called antigenic shift—a major change in the influenza A virus makeup. A pandemic is possible when a virus that has shifted can cause illness in

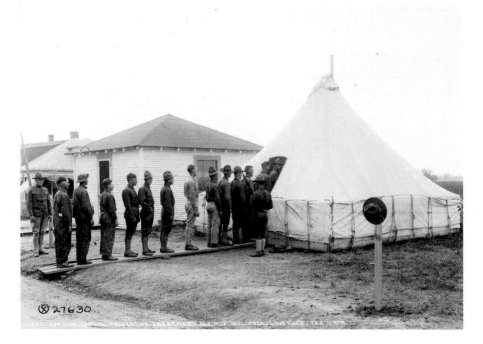

Love Field, Dallas, Texas. Preventative treatment against influenza. The line at the spraying station. *National Archives.*

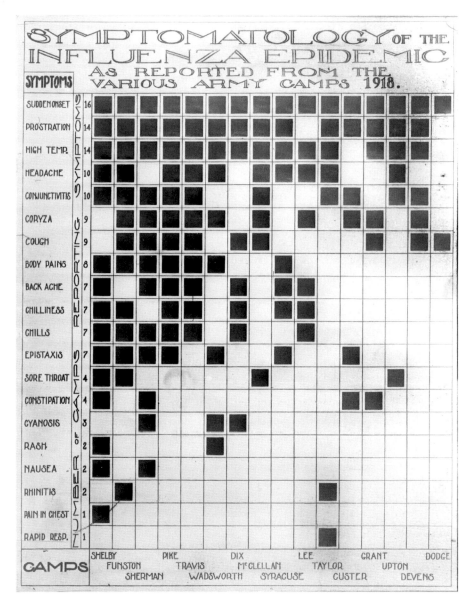

Symptomatology of the influenza epidemic as reported from the various army camps, 1918. The chart includes symptoms such as high temperature, headache, cough, body pains, rash, rhinitis, etc. *National Museum of Health and Medicine.*

people and can withstand sustained transmission, passing from person to person without losing its virulence. In these cases, most human populations would be considered naïve, meaning they've had no prior contact with this particular pathogen and are extremely susceptible.[26]

It's entirely possible that this is exactly what happened in early 1918 in rural Haskell County, Kansas. A group of pigs caught one or multiple viruses from another species. The viral strains underwent antigenic shift. They introduced themselves, mixed, mingled, and reproduced within the pigs' bodies before coming into contact with the farmers responsible for the animals' care. From person to person, household to household, region to region, the new variant viral strain spread, sickening and sometimes killing as it went, before taking a break and reemerging later that year, stronger than ever.

But how did this influenza strain, with a high morbidity but relatively low mortality rate, become so deadly later in the year? If it was indeed the same strain, as most scientists believe, it most likely went through a process called antigenic drift. While antigenic shift creates a major change in the virus—a change large enough to allow it to infect different species—antigenic drift is more subtle. When antigenic drift occurs, the influenza virus replicates within the hosts' cells and undergoes a number of genetic changes, or mutations. The virus's RNA, more susceptible to mutation than its DNA, changes. The hemagglutinin or neuraminidase proteins, or even both, become so different that the antibodies developed during previous exposure no longer offer protection against the virus. This can happen slowly, over one or more regular flu seasons, or quickly, over months or weeks. Most often, the changes are small and subtle, so people can be infected with a mutated version of an influenza strain they've had before and still have some level of immunity. In other instances, the changes are more dramatic, and the new, mutated strain is much more virulent and deadly than its earlier version.[27]

This is likely what happened in 1918. Over a few short weeks and months, the genetic makeup of the original viral strain changed and mutated as it passed through different populations, eventually growing stronger and deadlier. Like a bullied child, the young strain had two options: submit to the treatment thrown at it and keep its distance or focus on growing and strengthening, determined to take revenge when the time was right. It chose the latter.

PART II

OCTOBER 1918

Adieu, farewell earth's bliss!
This world uncertain is:
Fond are life's lustful joys,
Death proves them all but toys.
None from his darts can fly;
I am sick, I must die—
Lord, have mercy on us!

Rich men, trust not in wealth,
Gold cannot buy you health;
Physic himself must fade;
All things to end are made;
The plague full swift goes by;
I am sick, I must die—
Lord, have mercy on us!

—*Thomas Nashe, from "In Time of Pestilence"*

Chapter 4

TEN WHISTLES

On October 4, 1918, Michael Murtha, a forty-six-year-old miner in Butte, died of "bronchopneumonia and influenza."[28] An Irish immigrant, Murtha made his living in the depths of mines owned by the Anaconda Copper Mining Company. Like many single miners, he lived in a boardinghouse in Uptown Butte. At the time of his death, he called the Hegelton House his home, but he moved frequently. In the years prior, he had lived in places on East Broadway, on South Wyoming Street, and in Dublin Gulch. His transience wasn't uncommon for Butte's single miners. They would move often from mine to mine, house to house, always in search of the best deal. After a long shift underground, they might buy a drink (or a few), take in a match between amateur boxers in the back of a saloon, or perhaps visit the Red Light District. Some sent percentages of their earnings to family they'd left in other parts of the country or the world. Others saved for years to buy their families a small house they could call their own. They knew they'd never be as rich as the men who lived in the West Side mansions, but they still took pride in their work and enjoyed the meager fruits of their labor.[29]

Unfortunately, little else is known about Murtha's life. The circumstances of his death, though, would become all too familiar to hundreds of Butte's residents over the coming weeks. There is no record of exactly what Murtha felt during his fatal bout with influenza, but if it was like the experiences of millions of others around the world that autumn and winter, one can easily imagine how his last days may have unfolded.

Murtha's illness probably began with fatigue. This was different than the usual end-of-shift tiredness that Murtha would have felt upon each ascent from underground. Rather, the weariness was deep and crushing. His limbs felt heavy. His muscles and joints began to ache. As the sun began to go down over the western slopes, he made his way to the boardinghouse, growing increasingly dizzy. Perhaps he shared his bed with another miner. If so, this man was on the opposite shift, so Murtha probably hoped to get a few good hours of sleep before the other man got home and wanted his turn for some rest in the room's single bed. Murtha may have curled his long limbs in toward his torso in an effort to calm the shaking and shivering that jolted his body.

The next morning, Murtha was likely unable to get out of bed. The aches in his head and body would be worse than the day before, and he may have developed a dry cough that burned his already sore throat. He probably shook and shivered uncontrollably with fever, perhaps pulling blankets over himself one moment to ward off a chill, then throwing them on the floor the next as the heat became unbearable. Likely, his skin was slick with sweat, his clothing, pillow, and sheets drenched. He probably hadn't the energy to summon anyone to tell his shift boss he couldn't make it to work that day. In fact, it's likely the thought was far from his mind. It's more probable that the only things he could think about were how much his body hurt, how torched his fevered skin felt, and how his body felt it would split in half each time he coughed. If his roommate came home from his shift and tried to speak to Murtha, he almost certainly would have received no response. Perhaps he notified someone or just resigned himself to sleeping in another absent man's bed.

It's hard to estimate how long Murtha lay in bed. It may have been days or just hours; there is no record of when he first fell ill. It's likely, though, that he was pale and covered in a thin sheen of sweat. Perhaps he tossed and turned with fever, or maybe he lay motionless, a horrific, dry, hacking cough the only sign he was alive. Someone checking on him may have attempted to call a doctor. The doctor's advice probably would have been to have Murtha rest and take fluids and fresh air through an open window.

None of this would have helped Murtha, though, and before much more time had passed, his breathing would have changed as pneumonia invaded his lungs. Instead of rattling in his throat, Murtha's breaths would have sounded thick, like he was trying to breathe around a mouthful of water. The blood would have come next. Like later victims of pneumonia,

Murtha's coughs may have begun to produce a mouthful of bloody phlegm that spurted out of his mouth and ran down his chin. Perhaps it only happened once every twenty minutes or so. Maybe the blood ran each time he coughed. Witnesses would have been overwhelmed with terror and a powerful compassion. Perhaps they rolled the man on his side, hoping that would help him breathe easier. If on his back, he might choke on his own bloody sputum, so they would leave him on his side, even though it would cause a small stream of thin, watery blood to trickle from the corner of his mouth.

When witnesses found Murtha's body, what they would have seen was perhaps one of the most horrifying things tough, hardened miners—no strangers to violent injury and death—had ever comprehended. Though he was no longer breathing, it's possible that blood dribbled slowly from the corner of Murtha's purple lips and was dried over the side of his chin. Perhaps his eyes were closed. Maybe they had rolled back in his head, showing almost nothing but white. It's likely that the tip of his nose and his cheeks were tinged blue and his ears were purple, discolored by the lack of oxygen in his blood. He was completely still. His breath no longer struggled, rasped, and gurgled in his chest and throat. His fingers, bluish like his face, lay motionless, perhaps at his sides, but maybe clenched at his chest, as if he'd been trying to claw it open to get one last gasp of air.

The fatigue, aches, fever, chills, and dry cough that had been Murtha's first symptoms were hallmarks of influenza. The gurgling breaths and bloody phlegm signaled the beginning of pneumonia, which was the ultimate cause of death in many of the pandemic's mortalities. The blueish extremities were markers of cyanosis, a condition brought about by a lack of oxygen in the blood. Cyanosis was not only visibly horrifying but also a sign that death was imminent. Butte's doctors were familiar with the slow agony of tuberculosis, the feverish hacking of pneumonia, and even the aching coughs of influenza. But the pneumonia and influenza that killed Murtha was unlike any that the city's medical professionals had ever seen before. It struck suddenly and violently, and its presentation was horrifying.

By the time the contagion reached Butte in October 1918, doctors and health officials nationwide had finally determined they were most likely dealing with a strange and dangerous new type of influenza—one they'd never seen before. What they didn't know was how the disease could be defeated. This was a question they would spend the rest of the year attempting to answer. Over the next few months, physicians, public health professionals, and community leaders would fight battles over science, best health practices, and cultural differences. They would straddle the balance between disease control and civil liberties. They would institute community control measures, argue over their efficacy, recommend remedies, and, often simultaneously, disparage and praise those efforts.

Meanwhile, the disaster unfolding was worthy of ten piercing mine yard whistles.

Chapter 5

FIRST RESPONDERS

On September 27, 1918, exactly one week before Michael Murtha's death in Butte, sixteen-year-old Violet Paus of Scobey, in Montana's northeastern corner, died of a "cold" and "pleurisy."[30] Doctors later determined she was the state's first victim of the "Spanish influenza" that had been ravaging cities in the eastern United States. After its first initial flare-up in the spring, the illness had taken a bit of a break before coming back stronger than ever. At first confined mostly to military camps and places abroad, it was now widespread. Since August, influenza had meticulously been working its way across the country in a more violent form than ever. More Scobey residents, including Paus's mother, came down with the same illness that claimed Violet. Within a week, communities across Montana were waging their own battles with influenza. The virus followed railroad tracks, crisscrossing the state from city to city and disembarking at smaller communities in between. Influenza traveled rutted clay roads across the open prairie from towns and larger thoroughfares to small farms and ranches miles from the nearest neighbor. It journeyed through forests and over mountains, from one side of the Continental Divide to the other. On October 6, twenty-five soldiers at Fort Missoula, over five hundred miles from Scobey, were placed in quarantine "in the belief" that they suffered from "Spanish influenza."[31]

On October 7 alone, Dr. William F. Cogswell, at the offices of the Montana State Department of Health in Helena, received reports of five additional communities reporting influenza outbreaks. Dr. Cogswell, a native of Nova Scotia, Canada, had been practicing medicine in Montana since 1895, shortly after finishing his medical education at Dalhousie University in Halifax. His public health career began in 1908 as the Park County, Montana health officer. He was then appointed chairman of the Board of Entomology researching tick-borne spotted fever, and in 1912, he took over his position as the Montana State Board of Health executive secretary. Before October 7, 1918, though, Cogswell was not thinking about ticks or influenza but the Great War. His plan was to resign from the State Board of Health to join the Volunteer Medical Service Corps as part of the war effort. Cogswell perhaps recognized how his knowledge and experience in the prevention and mitigation of communicable disease might be of great use in the army. Perhaps he could help make this the first war in which disease didn't kill more soldiers than battle did. Other members of the Montana State Board of Health, however, also understood the importance of Cogswell's public health experience and expertise and were unwilling to let him go. They deferred accepting his resignation, effectively keeping him on the board for the duration of the pandemic and beyond. That decision, and Dr. Cogwell's consequent choice to act upon influenza immediately, would shape his entire career.[32]

Dr. Cogswell was unable to call a quorum of the State Board of Health on such short notice, so "acting under the authority given him" as a lead public health official for the State of Montana, he took it upon himself to issue "an emergency order requiring the closing of all schools, all public places of amusement, including theaters, and prohibiting the holding of public meetings in all communities where there have been outbreaks of the disease."[33] These were Cogswell's instructions for the general public. Public health officials and healthcare providers received additional orders. Doctors were to immediately report all cases and outbreaks to local public health departments, which in turn were to notify the state health department with case counts each week. Influenza patients were to remain isolated until recovery. Infection control measures in hospitals included screening all incoming patients for influenza, separating influenza patients from others, and disinfecting "all discharges from the nose and mouth of patients."[34] Cogswell had certainly seen and treated influenza before, and generally its appearance, especially in early autumn at the beginning of the usual influenza season, would be little cause for concern. Doctors would understand the disease was circulating in their communities, consider it as a diagnosis if symptoms warranted, and provide treatment accordingly. Early reports, though, helped Cogswell recognize that this infection was different. Influenza usually did not spread this far this quickly, infect such high numbers of people, and prove deadly to so many, especially those like Violet Paus and the soldiers at Fort Missoula who were in their prime health years. The sweeping action, Cogswell believed, was not only warranted but necessary.

About eighty miles to the south, Dr. Jed B. Freund was in his first month as secretary of the Butte–Silver Bow Board of Health. Freund was the son of Isadore D. Freund, one of Butte's most established and well-known physicians. The elder Freund, the son of German immigrants, received his medical education in Michigan, and by the turn of the twentieth century, he was part owner of the Murray Hospital (known as Murray and Freund's Hospital during the time he held interest there). Jed, along with his brother Raynor, followed Isadore into the medical profession. Jed attended West Point for two years before petitioning for and receiving an honorable discharge to attend medical school at the University of Michigan. Then he made his way back to Butte to practice. The morning of October 9, 1918 was the beginning of his baptism-by-fire into the world of public health.[35]

The Butte–Silver Bow Board of Health was joined that morning by Dr. Dan J. Donohue, Silver Bow County physician and president of the Montana State Board of Health. Donohue, a Wisconsin native, obtained his medical education at St. John's University in St. Cloud, Minnesota, and began his medical practice in Glendive, Montana, in 1900 after serving in the Spanish-American War. "Colonel Dan," as he was affectionately known in military circles, moved in 1915 to Butte, where, in addition to practicing medicine, he held a command position with the National Guard.[36]

Drs. Donohue and Freund and other public health officials quickly recognized that as Montana's most populous city, it was imperative that Butte institute the suggested measures as soon as the disease was identified within the city. The Montana State Health Department's guidance couldn't have arrived in Butte at a timelier moment. As county physician, Dr. Donohue had taken the first official reports of the disease just the day before—three cases and one death attributed to influenza. It's quite possible he was referring to Murtha, as his was the only official influenza death before October 10.

Three other Butte doctors present at the meeting reported patients with influenza "under treatment."[37] One of these doctors was Dr. Walter Colfax Matthews. Born in Brattleboro, Vermont, in 1869, Matthews received his medical education from the Baltimore College of Physicians and Surgeons and practiced medicine in New York and New England. After the death of his first wife in 1905, he made his way west, ultimately establishing himself in Butte. By 1918, he had remarried, had two daughters, was in private practice, and was serving as Butte's city physician. Influenza would make him a regular attendee of meetings of the Butte–Silver Bow Board of Health.[38]

Dr. Donohue presented the state's orders in their entirety, and after reviewing their own situation, Butte officials, certain they had an outbreak on their hands, took action. In order "to prevent widespread devastation by this contagious and deadly plague," the board made the order that "all schools, churches, theatres, moving picture shows, dance halls, parades, cabarets, and public dances, will be closed to the public, and bargain and bargain [sic] sales in stores and all public gatherings will be prohibited, until further notice."[39] The resolution passed unanimously. Arguments would have been fruitless; the orders from the state health department mandated those control measures.

Social distancing as a disease prevention technique was far from a new idea. In antiquity, lepers were separated from healthy populations as a means of preventing the spread of the disease. During the Middle Ages, wealthy residents fled cities for the rural countryside in hopes of avoiding the Black Death. The premise was simple: limit how often people come into unnecessary contact with others to limit the spread of disease. Butte's public health leaders hoped to slow and eventually stop the spread of influenza by reducing the number of people who congregated in one area. The city's residents could go to work, unless their workplace was included in the order, but little else. Canceling religious services and social events and eliminating other activities, like department store sales, that might bring large crowds together was the simplest way to avoid further contagion. If people stayed home, they had less chance of contracting influenza.

Such measures weren't without issues and critics, though. Forcing businesses to close meant a loss of revenue for proprietors and, depending on the establishment and situation, perhaps the entire community as well. Mandatory closures also raised questions of the rights regarding the free-market entrepreneur, religious liberty, and individual freedoms. Few people easily accepted disruptions to their daily lives and limitations and restrictions on their personal and professional activities, even—or perhaps especially—when the intervention came from a government agency. Then, as now, public health officials were given the difficult task of balancing civil liberties with public protection—a difficult task made even more trying in a diverse, independent-minded city like Butte.

Reverend Charles F. Chapman of the Butte Ministerial Association attended the Butte–Silver Bow Board of Health's October 11 meeting as

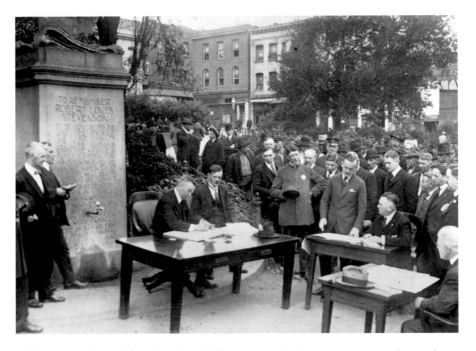

Police court officials of San Francisco holding a session in the open as a precaution against the spreading influenza epidemic. *National Archives.*

a representative of the city's religious communities. Reverend Chapman arrived in Butte in 1913 by way of North Platte, Nebraska, with his wife and four children. By 1918, he was in his mid-forties and had several years of ministerial experience.[40] His words to the board of health that morning illustrate that he was not only passionate but articulate as well. His argument immediately struck at the heart of the issue. The problem, Reverend Chapman argued, was not so much that churches must close their doors but that other places, namely saloons, were allowed to remain open. The decision to close churches and schools but allow saloons to stay in operation, the reverend stated, did not weigh the community's interests equally. He came to the board "not as a Minister only, but as an American Citizen. And on his rights as such, to ask equal rights to all, and special priveliages [*sic*] to none."[41] The board's decision to infringe upon the rights of some but not all, seemingly indiscriminately, didn't make sense. Of course, the reverend wanted his and other churches reopened, but in the absence of that objective, he simply desired fair application of the measures across all of the city's organizations and businesses.

The board of health certainly recognized and possibly even agreed with Reverend Chapman's argument, but its predicament was multilayered. Closing the saloons and pool halls would help slow the spread of disease. Due to round-the-clock shifts at the mines, these institutions were busy all hours of the day with regular customers and varying clientele. The city's saloons were a favorite after-work stop for the thousands of miners and other workers. They gathered to share news and information, especially important with the war overseas. It was much easier to close a house of worship, a place less frequently attended Monday through Saturday. It's possible the board members believed less public complaint would arise from closing those types of establishments as opposed to those visited regularly throughout the week with a devotion bordering on religious fervor by some. In the battle to protect the public's health while still maintaining the public's interest and respect, the board chose the conservative route. It preferred to keep the original order in "full force and effect until further notice."[42] One can only imagine Reverend Chapman's chagrin at the news that his and other places of worship should remain closed while saloons continued to operate.

Reverend Chapman was not alone in his dissent. Representatives from public and parochial schools also argued against the closures. The school board president stressed "co-operation in every way" with the board's endeavors to prevent influenza but believed it was "much better for the health of the community" to keep schools open because "sanitary conditions were much better in the Schools than on the Streets, and in the dirty alleys."[43] Children were exposed to more disease-causing germs on the streets than they were in school, education officials argued. Additionally, at school, children's comings and goings could be tracked and monitored. If schools closed, many children were unlikely to stay at home as officials intended. Instead, they would go out with their friends, walking the rail line to pick up pieces of dropped coal or wandering near the smelting stacks in search of overlooked bits of copper—popular pastimes for Butte youth in search of a few extra cents. Public school officials and parochial school representatives both agreed "the children would be better attending School, then [sic] on the streets."[44] But despite the ministrations of school officials, the board stayed firm. Though school faculty and administration may be vigilant about making sure the students practiced good health hygiene, in the end, closing schools minimized contact by disallowing children to congregate in closed rooms. "For the best interest of the Citizens and residents of Silver Bow County," the board concluded, the schools would remain closed.[45]

As the days wore on and Dr. Freund's daily updates on case numbers continued to rise, more businesses were deemed nonessential and required to close or limit hours. Cleanliness became a priority for usually dingy, dull Butte. Any businesses that were permitted to remain open were obligated to clean thoroughly each evening upon close, and staff members were required to wear masks. Daily, secretaries painstakingly disinfected offices, grocers scrubbed countertops, and waiters and waitresses all over Butte wore patches of gauze over their noses and mouths, removing them only to eat and drink and upon their returns home each day. Butte's streetcars, running across the hill between neighborhoods and mine yards, had to ensure proper ventilation. Drivers were asked to leave the windows open, even in the autumn mountain chill, to ensure passengers breathed fresh, clean air rather than the stale, recycled breath of other riders. A special "disinfective" was to be used when cleaning and sweeping sidewalks to help settle any dust that might carry disease-causing microbes. The mayor asked the fire chief to open hydrants and flush the streets, sending torrents of water and bits of street debris and garbage down the hill. For a few weeks, Butte—normally dusty and sooty, covered in layers of gray underneath the gray, smoke-filled sky that hung above—sparkled. There's probably no moment in history when Butte was physically cleaner than public health orders made it during the month of October 1918.[46]

For centuries, people have understood that disease can not only pass through human-to-human transmission but also by contact with an object that carries the infectious material—a fomite. In 1763, British general Jeffrey Amherst infamously passed smallpox to Native Americans united against the Crown during Pontiac's Rebellion by providing them with blankets that had been used in a smallpox hospital. In more recent history, it became common during the 2009 "swine flu" pandemic to find disinfecting wipes placed near grocery carts to cleanse their handles of any potentially infectious microbes. Butte health authorities well understood the risk of fomites. Libraries were closed so that "books taken and returned" did not "expose the Homes to the Influenza."[47] Public telephones were provided with disinfected covers, which were to be cleaned at least daily. Old phone directories were destroyed. Touching and moving those unnecessary books could spread any pathogens that had accumulated on them.[48]

As important as health officials believed cleaning was, social distancing remained the top priority. Dr. Freund had the unfortunate task of informing the city's seven undertakers, who in turn had to tell bereaved families, that large funerals would no longer be permitted. The crowds that gathered in

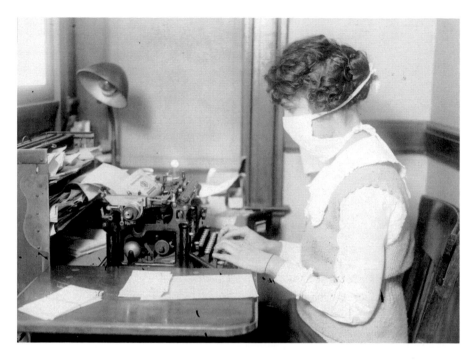

Above: A New York City typist wears a mask to protect against influenza in October 1918. This practice was common around the United States, including in Butte. *National Archives.*

Right: Streetcar windows were left open in an attempt to prevent the spread of influenza. This photo was taken in Cincinnati, but cities nationwide followed the practice. *National Archives.*

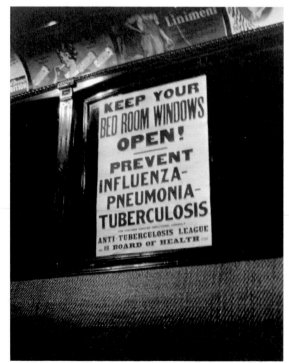

churches and even in the open air of cemeteries held just as much risk of spreading contagion as religious congregations and theatergoers. Priests could still say Mass and give absolution—acts required for Butte's majority Irish Catholic population—but until further notice, only immediate family would be allowed to attend funerals, even at graveside services. The undertakers agreed to "supply lists of relatives who will be the only persons admitted" to the services but were quick to point out that their duties during the services themselves would make it difficult for them to "prevent congestions."[49] In other words, the city's undertakers would inform the crowds who could attend services, but enforcing that measure was beyond their control. That was a task more suited for law enforcement.

Crowd control in general became a vital tool in mitigating contagion. Saloons could keep operating, but in moves aimed as much at social distancing as avoiding contagion through fomites, all tables and chairs were removed and drinks could not be sold over the bar. Instead, to dissuade patrons from gathering, only "package goods" were to be sold and carried away. No liquor was to be consumed on the premises.[50] Drs. Donohue, Freund, and Matthews began to believe "that the time had arrived when the Board of Health would be compelled to take drastic measures to combat the disease."[51]

These "drastic measures" were in regard to the control measures' enforcement. After the opposition brought so quickly by the school officials and Ministerial Association, board of health members undoubtedly expected more of the same from the public who would, perhaps, not be quite as polite or use the official channels to voice dissent. Early in October, board members engaged the sheriff's assistance "to use all means at his command to inforce [sic] the laws."[52] As premature as that strict action may seem, it became necessary as the months went by and Butte's residents became increasingly frustrated with the new requirements and restrictions placed upon them. Saloonkeepers worried over possible lost revenue. Tired, thirsty miners missed their daily glass of beer after hours spent working underground. More than a handful of establishments were accused of violating the new law. Barbers declined to wear their masks all day, every day. Dance halls held illegal gatherings. Butte residents refused to let influenza or authority stop them from living their daily lives. Less than two weeks after the sheriff was called upon to help with enforcement, board of health members agreed that "it was impossible to get the law enforced, that it had been tried and failed, and thought it was time to call on Military athorities [sic] to support the Board in their efforts to suppress the disease."[53] The board of health called upon the National Guard to "keep the crouds [sic] moving."[54] One can imagine that Butte looked like a city under siege. Its usually bustling streets were quiet and still, patrolled regularly by uniformed men ordering even the smallest groups to disperse.

In theory, Butte's disease control measures were well-intentioned public health practice. Despite their unpopularity and regular infractions, there's no telling how many people the practices saved from illness or death. But for many in Butte, they came too late. By October 15, health officials estimated there had been approximately twenty-three deaths attributable to influenza since the first of the month.[55] Mrs. Charles McDonald, thirty, died on October 16, the first of Butte's mortalities that fall and winter whose cause of death would be attributed solely to "Spanish Influenza."[56] Nearly each day when the board of health met, Dr. Freund had to report increasingly larger numbers of influenza cases and deaths. Finally, on October 21, Dr. Freund reported that "Spanish influenza was on the increase but no definate [sic] figures could be given, for the Doctors were over worked and had no time to report."[57] Freund and other health officials believed the true number of cases was much higher than officially counted. There were far too few doctors for the number of patients, and some residents probably hadn't even attempted to notify a physician. Dozens of Butte residents, the board of health believed, sickened and probably died without ever seeing a doctor. There was no way to accurately estimate the true morbidity rate. Meanwhile, the deaths continued, unabated, for the rest of the month. On average, eight Butte residents died of influenza each day in October.[58]

Chapter 6

TREATING THE "MOST PECULIAR DISEASE"[59]

Throughout the autumn of 1918, the Butte–Silver Bow Board of Health seemed to place its focus on prevention measures in the battle against influenza. Indeed, this was public health's primary responsibility—and continues to be today—in such an event: mitigate the spread of disease by investigating the cause, ascertain those who may be at risk, and establish measures to stop the spread. Treatment of an illness or condition was, and is, primarily left to healthcare providers. This is not to say that public health agencies didn't play a role in treating communicable diseases. In many instances, treatment was a cooperative activity, especially in the early days of public health, when doctors were the primary members of local health departments and boards of health.[60] Since public health's inception, local health departments have provided guidance and resources to healthcare providers regarding the best available treatment methods and options in cases of communicable disease. Public health's strength has always lay in delivering information and resources for dealing with multi-patient situations, like an outbreak, epidemic, or pandemic. Where physicians typically have had a single-patient perspective, public health's focus has been on the community as a whole.

Additionally, one of public health's largest assets was, and is, its knowledge of available resources and ability to mobilize them. When it comes to requesting additional resources—including medical supplies, facilities, large quantities of medication, and human resources—hospitals and healthcare providers could rely on the channels available through public health. In 1918, the Butte–Silver Bow Board of Health called upon this store of knowledge and connections to help supply the city's healthcare providers with all of those resources.

One of the first things physicians came face to face with during the pandemic was the frustrating and devastating conclusion that, most of the time, there was very little they could do to treat a patient suffering from influenza. In the decades leading up to 1918, medical science had made enormous strides. Germ theory was widely accepted by the 1890s, replacing the theory of miasma, which held that disease was essentially caused by "bad air." According to miasma theory, poisonous vapors in the air caused disease. Scientists had learned to identify various bacteria under the microscope, and the first virus was identified in the 1890s. By the early 1900s, blood type had been discovered and many different vaccines developed.

The science of disease itself had evolved. Doctors no longer practiced bloodletting, the barbaric treatment of choice for centuries in which physicians surgically opened veins to purge "bad blood" and any disease-causing agents it may carry. Surgeons now used anesthetic when performing surgery. Physicians followed Joseph Lister's work on sterilization and antiseptics, helping to prevent infection. Yet diagnostic ability outpaced that of treatment. Doctors observed and reported clinical findings, ordered lab tests, and conducted autopsies, all in the name of identifying a malady's culprit. Even here, though, science proved insufficient with influenza in 1918.

Contemporary medical science seemed to have a crisis of identity regarding influenza itself. In 1907, a chapter on influenza in Dr. William Osler's expansive *Modern Medicine* identified a number of different clinical types of influenza, including those of the "circulatory system, of the genito-urinary system, of the joints, and of the skin."[61] Of course, influenza's usual target was the respiratory system, but the symptoms perceived in influenza sufferers during outbreaks and epidemics of the nineteenth and early twentieth centuries varied. This led the day's leading medical authorities to speculate widely not only on the disease's clinical presentation but its treatment as well. After all, urinary tract conditions are treated much differently than bone and joint or cardiovascular issues.

Another problem was that the 1918 strain of influenza was much different from any contemporary physicians had ever seen. Along with the violent, agonizing deaths so many patients suffered, doctors were astounded by the illness's speedy progression. "Do you know this is the most peculiar disease I have ever seen?" a hospital administrator in Glasgow, Montana, noted. The

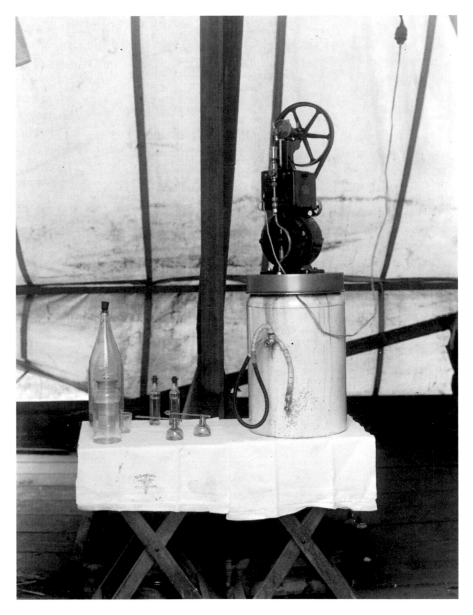

Spraying machine, preventive treatment against influenza, Love Field, Texas. *National Archives.*

disease often advanced so quickly, she continued, that "some persons hardly know they are sick until they're dying."[62] Yale professor and epidemiologist Charles-Edward Amory Winslow reported "a number of cases where people were perfectly healthy and died within twelve hours."[63] Influenza didn't usually act like that, contemporary medical professionals agreed. Modern medicine was baffled. In the pandemic's early days, physicians labeled the disease bronchopneumonia or respiratory infection. None of the usual treatments for those illnesses worked, though. Perhaps the malady was something rarer: typhus, dengue fever, or even a reappearance of the bubonic plague—the "Black Death" of Medieval Europe. One Chicago physician believed that "the present war diet," especially reduced sugar consumption, caused the illness.[64] A few believed the illness was part of a German operation to win the war—an early twentieth-century form of bioterrorism.[65]

Specialists in the new field of medical laboratory science got involved. Laboratories, both private and affiliated with public hospitals and universities, began studying specimens collected from the disease's victims. Influenza is a filterable virus, meaning it is too small to be filtered through most of the laboratory equipment available to scientists in 1918. The virus is much smaller than most bacteria; hence, it's more difficult to isolate. The influenza virus wasn't identified until the 1930s, and the strain that caused the 1918 pandemic wasn't discovered until the late 1990s. What 1918 researchers did find in their samples was evidence of *Pfeiffer's bacillus*—a bacterium discovered during an influenza outbreak in 1892. German physician and bacteriologist Richard Pfeiffer reported isolating a rod-shaped bacterium in each influenza sample he had examined. *Pfeiffer's bacillus* was difficult to grow and stain, making it hard to study, but to Pfeiffer and his contemporaries, it provided a clear, scientifically based hypothesis for the cause of influenza. However, later researchers also isolated *Pfeiffer's bacillus* in specimens taken from victims of diseases like pertussis (whooping cough), varicella (chickenpox), and measles. In retrospect, it seems obvious that *Pfeiffer's bacillus* was not the cause of influenza but a relatively common comorbidity. To desperate researchers, doctors, and their patients, though, it offered answers where no other explanation existed.[66]

Today, medical science believes *Pfeiffer's bacillus* causes *Haemophilus influenzae*, or *H. influenzae*. Despite its name, *H. influenzae* does not cause influenza but is responsible for illnesses like meningitis and bloodstream infections and is one of the most common causes of pneumonia. It's probable, then, that the *Pfeiffer's bacillus* isolated in the 1918 specimens came from patients who had already or would soon develop pneumonia.

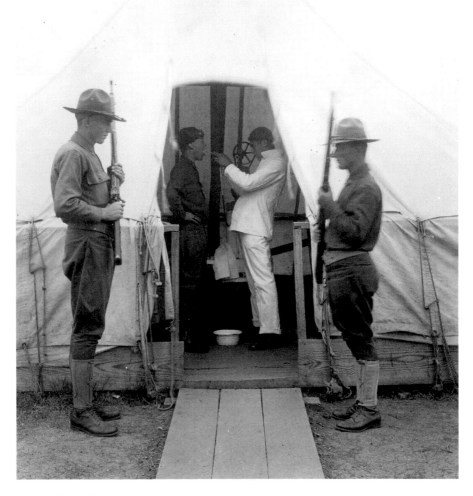

Love Field, Dallas, Texas. Preventive treatment against influenza, spraying the throat.
National Archives.

Had antibiotics existed, they would not have helped with influenza—a viral illness—but could have treated the invasion of *Pfeiffer's bacillus* and perhaps staved off the deadly pneumonia.[67]

Let down by the medical science the past decades' progress had led them to place so much faith in, doctors grasped at straws. They were unable to treat the disease's cause and struggled to manage the symptoms. Some treatments were more successful than others. Acetylsalicylic acid, named aspirin by the Bayer Company in 1899, was given for fever and pain, which certainly helped manage symptoms to some extent. Epinephrine was given to those suffering from pneumonia, probably in hopes of relaxing the airways. This was less successful. Patients with cyanosis were given oxygen through masks (helpful) or had it injected under their skin (less helpful). Some patients were given quinine. Many of their symptoms—high fever, chills, aches—resembled those of malaria, so doctors thought maybe the same treatment would work. It didn't.[68]

The United States Public Health Service offered "Uncle Sam's Advice on Flu," syndicated in newspapers around the nation and phrased in a way that made it very clear to Americans just how serious this illness was: "Coughs and Sneezes Spread Diseases," a subheading read, "As Dangerous as Poison Gas Shells."[69] For months, Americans on the homefront had heard about the horrors of the invisible and deadly vapors of chlorine and mustard gas—how they blistered the skin, caused sneezing and turned the throat raw, how the victims coughed up blood and struggled to breathe. This threat—this invisible germ—they were now told, was just as deadly and should be taken just as seriously. The illness, the guidance stated, was so dangerous, in part, because of its proclivity to take one by surprise. The symptoms may be similar to that of a cold except in their sudden onset and severity.

> *In most cases a person taken sick with influenza feels sick rather suddenly. He feels weak, has pains in the eyes, ears, head or back, and may be sore all over. Many patients feel dizzy, some vomit....In appearance one is struck by the fact that the patient looks sick. His eyes and the inner side of his eyelids may be slightly "bloodshot," or "congested," as the doctors say. There may be running from the nose, or there may be some cough.*[70]

Besides the patient's symptoms and appearance, diagnosis could be made by "examination of the patient's blood." This was imprecise, however, and the United States Public Health Service was hopeful that further research by "the National Research Council and the United States Hygienic Laboratory will furnish a more certain way in which individual cases of this disease can be recognized."[71] In other words, medical science was still playing catch-up. Healthcare and public health professionals understood that this disease was contagious and deadly, but exactly how to recognize it, outside of identifying the clinical symptoms, was still a guessing game.

The United States Public Health Service admitted the disease's cause was also elusive. *Pfeiffer's bacillus* may be the responsible agent, they reported, as "bacteriologists who have studied influenza epidemics in the past have found in many of the cases" that particular microbe. However, the federal officials continued, "in other cases of apparently the same kind of disease there were found *pneumococci*, the germs of lobar pneumonia. Still others have been caused by *streptococci*, and by others [*sic*] germs with long names."[72] *Pfeiffer's bacillus* could be responsible, but so might other bacteria. Or perhaps it could be some combination of those. And it remained that the cause could be something else entirely—something that the day's brightest medical minds had yet to discover.

But the United States Public Health Service was quick to reassure, "no matter what particular kind of germ causes the epidemic," the spread could be prevented by ill persons staying home to avoid "scattering the disease far and wide." In fact, "no one but the nurse should be allowed in the room," and those nurses should guard against catching the disease themselves by "wearing a simple fold of gauze or mask while near the patient."[73] As far as patient care, those who had fevers and headaches "should be given water to drink, a cold compress to the forehead, and a light sponge." Patients were advised to guard against medicines unless they came from a doctor. "It is foolish," the advice continued, "to ask the druggist to prescribe and may be dangerous to take the so-called 'safe, sure, and harmless' remedies advertised by patent medicine manufacturers."[74]

This warning against patent medicines emerged from a real contemporary problem. Through the centuries, medical practitioners have devoted their entire lives to finding remedies for human ailments of all symptoms and severities. Early on, their searches were experimentation—journeys in trial and error that often caused more harm than good or were even deadly. Mercury didn't cure syphilis but slowly poisoned the patient. Mixtures given to induce vomiting and relieve the body of bad "humors" left the sufferer even weaker. At best, the remedies did nothing, simply leaving the patient in a state similar to before he or she had used the drug. A few of these early experiments, though, did amount to something successful. Willow bark helped to alleviate pain and swelling and was synthesized to create aspirin. Opium would also relieve pain, leading to the eventual development of narcotic painkillers. Cinchona bark, used to quell shivering, contained quinine, which was found to be a successful treatment for malaria. Researchers discovered that their new knowledge of chemistry could change these "natural" remedies into something even more powerful. Technology fused with naturopathy, and by the twentieth century, a new type of pharmaceutical paradise was created. A novel drug was available to cure any ailment that one might suffer.

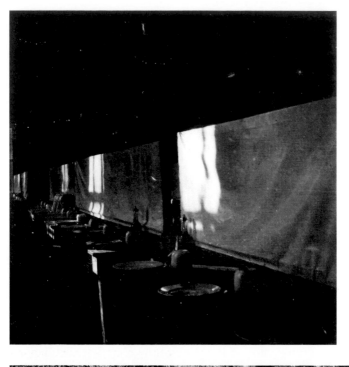

Partitions out of oilcloth hung the length of the tables at Fort Thomas, Kentucky, during the influenza epidemic to prevent germs traveling across in the event of accidental sneezing. *National Archives.*

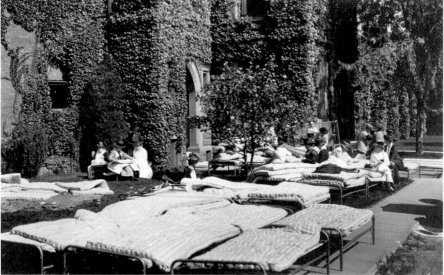

American Red Cross activities in Middletown, Connecticut. Emergency hospital equipment is being inspected by the committee of the Middlesex chapter. This equipment was sent to Wesleyan University at the outbreak of the influenza epidemic. *National Archives.*

However, the legitimacy of many of these "wonder drugs" was questionable at best. With no regulating body to test and license each medication, the patent medicine industry was born. The boom year was 1918. The makers of Sozodont, a tooth powder that included calcium carbonate, magnesia, glycerin, water, and alcohol on its list of ingredients, claimed that it would keep teeth and gums strong and kill the germs that caused influenza. E.W. Grove's Laxative Bromo Quinine would help ease the symptoms of influenza by maintaining bowel regularity. A mask slathered with Kolyos, another oral care aid, would "Fight Spanish Influenza when Exposed to Infection." Influ-Balm also claimed to prevent influenza. If one did come down with the disease, though, he or she could use Men-Tho-Eze for "relief in twenty minutes."[75] Exactly how each of these concoctions worked to prevent or cure influenza was left vague in the advertising. Likely, some of the remedy-makers themselves were unsure how their own wares worked. All swore that their medicine made a difference, and some truly believed in their product. Others were mere peddlers and quacks, exploiting the public's fear to make money. The truth was that no maker could guarantee its cure. If medical science couldn't explain and treat influenza, how could an amateur chemist? The legacy of the patent medicine industry lived beyond the pandemic, though. Lysol and Vick's Vapo-Rub, household names now, are just two products that owe their popularity to the fight against influenza in 1918.

Medical science refused to be waylaid by the prevalence of magical cures and patent medicines. By 1918, researchers had developed a number of successful vaccines—rabies, typhoid, and diphtheria, as well as an antitoxin for diphtheria, just to name a few. Many doctors and scientists believed there was no reason one of those vaccines wouldn't work to combat influenza. Drug companies touted their stock vaccines of "undisclosed composition" in the fight against the flu. After all, if science was unsure what caused the illness, how could they be sure these things wouldn't work? Scientists worked on developing a vaccine that would specifically target *Pfeiffer's bacillus*. In one extreme example, University of Pittsburgh researchers developed, tested, and distributed a vaccine to the Red Cross for use on humans against *Pfeiffer's bacillus* all in the span of one week. Many patients given these various *Pfeiffer's bacillus* vaccines reported positive results. If the vaccine did, in fact, work, it's likely that its primary use was not in preventing influenza but the pneumonia that often followed and proved so deadly.[76]

In Butte, Dr. Freund took notice of the reports he'd read about the success of a vaccine "used in the Ship Yards and Navy, with a great success."[77] He petitioned the Butte–Silver Bow Board of Health to purchase a small trial amount. It agreed to two hundred doses. The county jail's population and patients in the county hospital, board members believed, provided the perfect test groups for the vaccine. On November 3, Drs. Freund and Donohue reported that they'd witnessed "good results" from the eighty-seven county jail inmates who had received the vaccine. Likewise, the results coming from the county hospital were also "very good," though exactly what that meant is unclear.[78] Drs. Freund and Donohue didn't indicate exactly how the vaccine had helped—if it prevented illness or mitigated symptoms. Meanwhile, in Helena, Dr. Cogswell sent the state's "chemist" to Rochester, Minnesota, possibly to the Mayo Clinic, to "investigate the merits of the vaccine."[79] Though the chemist heartily believed in the vaccine's effectiveness as a preventative, the state board of health did not endorse its use. The exact reason for that decision is unknown. Perhaps there were simply too many unknowns about the vaccine itself—its composition, how it worked, and its effects on the human body—for state health officials to risk trying it on Montanans, desperate as they were.[80]

Meanwhile, the general guidance on fighting infection and recovering from the illness was as vague as the ingredient list on a patent medicine. A few "Hints for Influenza Victims" were to:

> *Open all windows in your bedroom and keep them open at all times, except in rainy weather.*
> *Cleanse nose and throat with any mild antiseptic, as weak solution of salt and soda, listerine, glycothymolin, etc.*
> *Take medicine to open the bowels freely.*
> *Take some nourishing food, such as milk, egg-and-milk, or broth every four hours.*
> *Stay in bed until a physician tells you that it is safe to get up.*[81]

While this advice certainly wouldn't have exacerbated most influenza cases, it probably did very little to actually help slow or stop the progression of the disease. Medical professionals had simply determined that there was little they could do to help patients besides keeping them comfortable.

Comfort care was not within the realm of doctors, trained to treat the causes of illness with proven scientific remedies, but of nurses. The war in Europe made this type of care exceedingly difficult to come by, though. Around the nation, resources were allocated first toward the war effort. This included medical personnel. Dr. Cogswell was far from

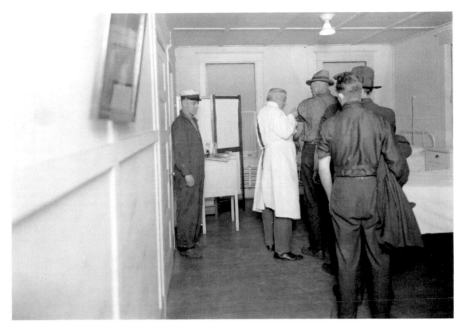

The military provided "flu serum injections" to service members. This photo was taken in Seattle. *National Archives.*

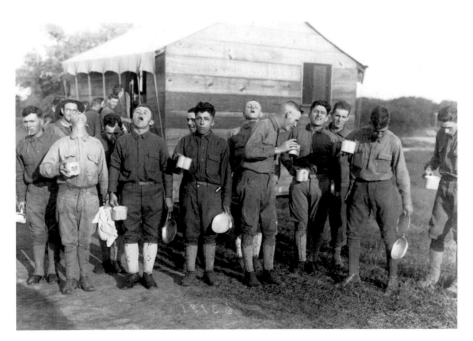

Soldiers gargle with salt and water at the end of the workday at Camp Dix, New Jersey. This practice was thought to help prevent influenza. *National Archives.*

being alone in his wish to join the service. A full 30 percent of American physicians left their regular practice to join the military effort, and most of America's nurses had already been pressed into service by the military and were serving overseas or in stateside camps. The army counted approximately 21,500 nurses in its ranks, the navy another 1,700. Consequently, many stateside cities and communities were left incredibly shorthanded regarding medical professionals and support staff to care for their needs. To help increase the number of trained caregivers, the Nurses' Association in Helena upped the weekly wages 25 percent, to $35 per week and "$40 a week for contagious cases." In this case, more risk equaled more reward. They also increased nurses' leave time from two to three hours for every twenty-four hours worked.[82]

The pay and leave increases were well deserved. The nurses who answered the call at home to fight influenza faced as much risk in 1918 as those sent overseas with the army. Before October was over, Murray Hospital had lost two of its nurses to influenza. Blanche Cook, twenty-two, and Alberta Van Vranken, twenty-eight, were both senior nursing students at Murray Hospital when they made "the supreme sacrifice—doing their duty so that others might live." Though both young women were "earnest students and were well equipped to help fight the dread malady…they were not equal to resisting the iron clutch of the ruthless epidemic." Both were remembered with fondness and respect by their teacher and colleagues.[83]

The Red Cross took an active role in providing care and other invaluable services above and beyond its mask-making project during the fall and winter of 1918. Dr. Freund placed the management of the city and county nurses under the Red Cross's jurisdiction to help aid the communication process and streamline the nursing response. The Red Cross also did what it could to ensure the health of Butte's more vulnerable and disadvantaged residents— the hundreds living in poverty. It started a voluntary service, asking private citizens to volunteer as "visiting nurses." "There are not sufficient nurses in Butte to meet this emergency….Offer your services as a visiting nurse," the Red Cross advertisement read. "Experience not necessary," it added in parentheses, illustrating the city's dire need for caregivers.[84] Training was helpful, but the largest need was for caring, compassionate individuals willing to sit at their neighbors' bedsides and keep them as comfortable as possible. Many of Butte's residents stepped up to answer the call. By early November, between fifty and sixty of the city's teachers had volunteered their time to serve as nurses while the schools were closed. So many teachers volunteered that the reopening of Butte's schools was delayed, as it was not "fair to the

School Children of Butte, that these teachers be permitted to resume their work at this time" because they "have ben [sic] exposed to the disease."[85] The care of Butte's sick residents and the protection of its vulnerable children took precedence over education.

Facilities were also in short supply. On October 23, Dr. Freund expressed concern that, even with incidences of influenza "on the decrease," there were still many cases that required "special attention" to fully recover.[86] These sufferers needed more care than could be provided at home, yet all beds at both the county and privately owned hospitals were full. Drs. Freund and Matthews joined forces with Trevor Bowen of Butte's Red Cross chapter to establish a temporary emergency hospital for the care of influenza patients.

In his work with the Red Cross, Bowen had already established emergency hospitals in other neighboring communities. Butte's larger size and needs presented a new challenge. The first was location. The board of health weighed the benefits and drawbacks of different facilities. Hotelier James T. Finlen generously volunteered his Uptown Butte property as a possible location. "I will absolutely close up the place and turn it over to some responsible authority," Finlen stated. "I'm convinced that something drastic must take place to curb the spread of the epidemic," he added.[87] His hotel could "accommodate at least 200 patients," Finlen stated, adding that more cots could be placed in the café area, and hospital staff could use the kitchen to prepare meals. All he asked in return was that the authorities make responsible use of his property and ensure it wasn't "abused" and that it was returned in good condition.[88] "Use all we have, ask us for anything we have and make the sick well," Finlen concluded.[89] His offer illustrates the concerns running through not just the city's community of health professionals but its entire citizenry. His hotel was one of the finest in the city, and he was willing to close it to paying travelers for the sole use of influenza sufferers—a gesture that illustrates the care the people of Butte felt for their city and fellow residents. Butte was suffering—physically, emotionally, financially—and its people were willing to do whatever they could to help end the sorrow.

Despite Finlen's generous offer, Bowen and Drs. Freund and Matthews ultimately decided on Washington Junior High as the best place for this "Isolation Hospital," as the school was "considered in every way Sanitary and the best place available for the purpose of caring for emergency cases."[90] Here, patients could be easily kept away from their healthy friends and neighbors and remain accessible to medical staff—a twofold approach aimed at slowing the spread of infection and providing care for the city's neediest residents.

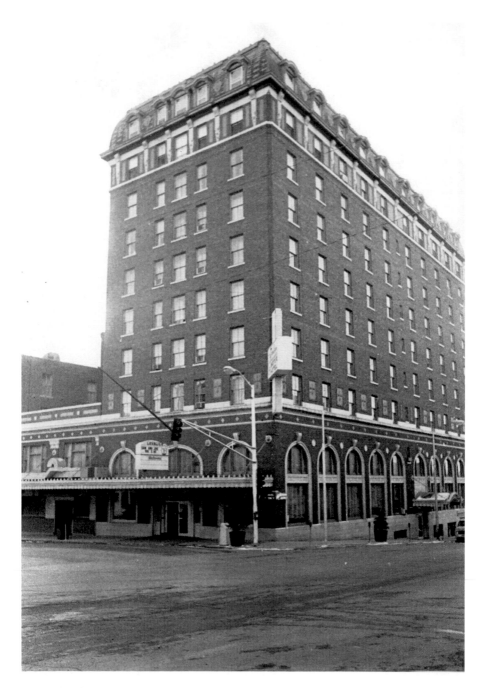

The Finlen Hotel at 120 East Broadway. This photo was taken after James Finlen rebuilt his hotel in the 1920s. *Butte–Silver Bow Public Archives.*

Determining a facility was just the first step in creating an operational hospital. Patient care required staff and equipment. Patients needed food, beds to rest in, and clean linens. The hospital needed nurses, cooks, and janitorial staff to fulfill these needs. Bowen and Drs. Freund and Matthews were given authority to purchase whatever supplies necessary to set up the facility and provide patient care. They were fortunate enough, Bowen reported, to have the high school's Domestic Science Department volunteer to take responsibility for preparing patients' meals, but that still left them with many other concerns. Today, the federal government can provide the equipment necessary to establish a temporary emergency medical facility. It can deliver beds, linens, medications, and other basic supplies to help respond to pandemic influenza or other disasters in which needs outstrip local resources. This option didn't exist in 1918's public health system, though. Officials in Butte and Silver Bow County rallied to care for their own. By county edict, up to $10,000 in emergency funds could be spent

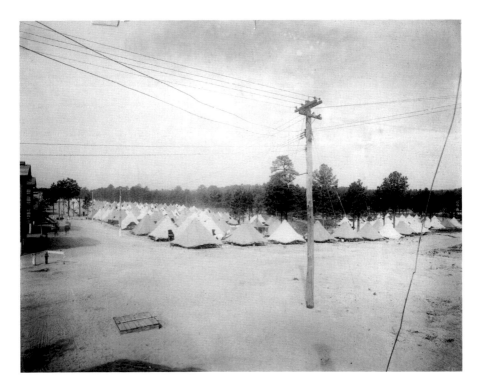

Enlisted men's tents during the influenza epidemic, Camp Jackson, Columbia, South Carolina. *National Museum of Health and Medicine.*

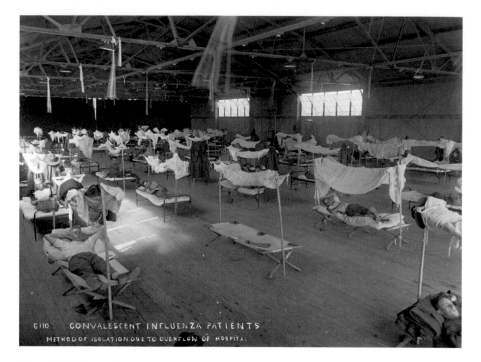

Eberts Field, Lonoke, Arkansas. Convalescent influenza patients are seen in this method of isolation due to the overflow at the hospital. *National Archives.*

on the hospital, and Bowen pledged the Red Cross's support in paying any additional expenditures. In another show of Butte's generosity, the Anaconda Copper Mining Company, the city's largest employer, volunteered to supply beds and linens and even an ambulance to transport patients. To admit a patient, doctors were instructed to "telephone No. 750 and an ambulance will call for them [patients]." Ill persons without a physician's referral but still seeking "medical attention should also call 750 and a nurse" would come to their residence.[91] Within two days, the emergency hospital was open and holding thirty-eight patients. Additional beds were requested to help with continued admissions. By the time another two days had passed, the hospital was operating at capacity.[92]

The facility, Bowen proudly reported, was "a great help" to the health department.[93] The emergency hospital took the strain off doctors struggling to visit patients all over the city and report back with accurate case numbers. Care was more efficient, saving nurses and doctors time and decreasing the period patients had to wait to be seen. The Red Cross's efforts also ensured that the impoverished or those who could not get a doctor to visit would still be seen by a healthcare worker. The Washington Emergency Hospital remained operational throughout October, November, and much of December, increasing its capacity as the weeks wore on. By November 29, Dr. Freund reported the hospital "was equipped to handle 200 patients."[94]

Throughout the pandemic's first weeks, Butte's doctors, nurses, and public health professionals used every tool at their disposal—human resources, equipment, knowledge—to fight the disease. They understood the severity and urgency of the situation. Many of the people of Butte, however, did not. In mid-October, two Butte residents returned to the city after a trip to Seattle, Washington with a warning. In Seattle, they reported, "the only place not closed...is the cemetery." Influenza had rendered the rest of the city as deserted as a ghost town. "At first people [in Seattle] laughed," the duo told the *Butte Miner*. "Now they are alarmed, and fear is increased by the constant presence of the hearse." The people of Butte, they cautioned, ought to take notice. "Some people in Butte are laughing; they are jeering but before the attack has ceased they will understand the gravity of the situation."[95] They were correct. In October, many of Butte's residents may not have taken the comparison between influenza and "poison gas shells" seriously. Many families, though, would come to understand the increasing "gravity of the situation" all too well.

Chapter 7

THE INDISCRIMINATE KILLER

he sick and dying were miners, waiters, bartenders, housewives, maids, railroad men, farmers, grocers, brewers, and nurses. They came from different backgrounds, social circles, and economic circumstances, but influenza leveled the playing field. Several instances in October made it apparent that no one in Butte was completely safe from the disease.

John O'Meara was the epitome of the American dream. Born in Ireland, O'Meara immigrated at the age of fifteen and went to work as a tool boy in the Alice Mine. His determination, work ethic, and "remarkable ability" got him steadily promoted, first to shift boss, then foreman, and finally mine superintendent. Nearly twenty years after his arrival in Butte, though, O'Meara left his successful mining career to manage Centennial Brewing. Later, he sold his holdings in Centennial and moved to Olympia Brewing. The two companies later merged, and he reclaimed his title as Centennial's manager. With his success in business also came civic recognition. O'Meara served as president of the Butte chapter of the Ancient Order of Hibernians for six years, was a member of the Butte Country and Silver Bow Clubs, and had been actively engaged in volunteer work "aiding the nation" since war had been declared in 1917. By 1918, John O'Meara and his wife, Sarah, had five children—four daughters and a son. Sadie and Virginia, the two youngest girls, still lived at home in Butte with their parents.[96]

But influenza didn't care how successful the O'Mearas were. On the morning of October 24, three hearses sat outside 307 West Granite Street, in the heart of one of Butte's most upscale neighborhoods. A crowd of hundreds watched the hearses leave for the triple funeral of John, Sarah, and twenty-two-year-old Sadie. John and Virginia, the youngest O'Meara child, had fallen ill with influenza in early October. Sarah and Sadie worked day and night nursing the two, and their efforts seemed to pay off when John and Virginia recovered. Influenza wasn't done with the O'Mearas, though. Whether from their exhaustive efforts, proximity to infection, or a combination of both, Sarah and Sadie both took ill. In a matter of days, they were both dead of the disease they'd saved John and Virginia from. When people learned about their deaths, "hundreds of Butte friends were shocked. She [Mrs. O'Meara] had been well only a few days before."[97]

A double funeral was scheduled for October 23, enough time, John hoped, for his oldest children to travel home from school. They arrived in Butte the day before the funeral, in time to witness influenza bring down their weak and grief-stricken father once again. John O'Meara died in the early morning hours of October 23, 1918. The double funeral was postponed a day, and a triple funeral was held in St. Patrick's Church on the twenty-fourth. The O'Mearas' success and prestige merited the family's tragic saga long stories in two Butte dailies, but it was not "the most sweeping devastation which influenza caused to any one family," as the *Butte Miner* claimed.[98]

Just weeks after the O'Meara funeral, the Mueller family tragedy began. After moving to the city from Wisconsin in the early 1880s, the Muellers quickly rose up the social and economic ranks of Butte society. Henry Mueller, the family patriarch, and his wife, Margaret, had five children, all of whom spent most of their childhoods in Butte. Henry started the Centennial Brewing Company and was elected the city's mayor in 1892. The eldest son, Arthur, attended Notre Dame and then returned to Butte, married Kathryn Sullivan, and had two sons, Arthur Jr. and Charles. Arthur and his brother Walter took over as president and treasurer, respectively, of Centennial Brewing after the death of their father in 1908.

Their work at Centennial and influenza seemed intertwined. Both Arthur and Walter served as pallbearers at the O'Meara funeral; John had been the brewery's manager, and the families shared the same social circles. Within six weeks, both Arthur and Walter had also become victims of influenza. Arthur died on November 27, after a weeklong battle with the disease, and Walter succumbed on December 9.

But there were many other families the *Miner* could have given the dubious honor it bestowed on the O'Mearas. Patrick Sullivan, an Irish-born miner, lived with his family in Centerville. A number of the city's largest mines dotted the areas in and around this neighborhood: the Mountain

Consolidated and the Bell Diamond sat within Centerville, and the infamous North Butte properties (the Granite Mountain and the Speculator) lay just to the northeast. Centerville's small houses sat high on the hill's dirty, crooked streets and were a far cry from the orderly mansions in the O'Mearas' neighborhood a few blocks to the southwest.

In late October, probably about the same time as the O'Meara triple funeral, thirty-four-year-old Patrick fell ill. If his illness followed the usual course, his head and body ached, and he wanted nothing more than to lie down and rest. But Patrick probably knew he had to make his shift at the mine. Production was high, men needed jobs, and he knew that there were men ready to take his place if he missed a shift. He may have wiped cold sweat from his brow while simultaneously pulling a long-sleeved shirt over his shaking shoulders to ward off the chill of fever. Then Patrick would have developed a cough that wouldn't go away but grew stronger, coming from deep in his midsection. Perhaps he gave up on going to work and instead tried to get into bed as the coughing fits doubled him over. Patrick developed pneumonia, and his family would have watched with horror as his previously dry coughs began to produce a frightening amount of mucousy phlegm. If he tried to catch it in a cloth, it may have come away from his face tinged with blood.

Patrick's fourteen-month-old son Peter probably fell ill at about this time. Patrick may have been too sick to witness his son's suffering. He died on October 26, and the baby followed a day later, his small body completely overwhelmed by the powerful virus. Influenza wasn't done with the Sullivan household, though. Patrick's wife and four other children also fell ill with influenza and were taken to the emergency hospital. Five-year-old Michael died on November 2. Patrick Sullivan's cousin Patrick Casey, "regarded as one of the strongest men employed on the hill, of magnificent physique and never ill a day," died of influenza on the same day as young Peter. Casey's sister Nellie Sullivan owned a boardinghouse and, though she was also ill, continued about her chores. Word of her brother's death reached Nellie as she was preparing a meal for her boarders. The shock and strain was too much, and "she collapsed and died within two hours."[99]

Several families experienced tragedy on the scale of the O'Mearas and Sullivans as autumn turned to winter in Butte. Twenty-five-year-old Emma Duffy died on October 18; within five days, her husband, Frank, twenty-nine, died as well. Daniel Sheedy, a miner working at the Speculator, died on October 24, the same day as his eight-year-old son and namesake. Frances and Rose McLaughlin, both twenty-one, died just a day apart in the last week of the month. In October alone, dozens of Butte families mourned a son, daughter, husband, or wife simultaneously or had no chance to attempt recovery from a loss before suffering another.[100]

Viruses don't think. They don't reason. They don't differentiate between race, class, or religion. All they need is a host. While this virus took over whatever hosts were available, it grew apparent as the weeks wore on that some groups of people were more desirable hosts than others. Influenza may not have discriminated, but it did have preferences. Its preferred tastes, though, wouldn't be fully recognized until later.

PART III

NOVEMBER 1918

And I looked, and there before me was a pale horse! Its rider was named Death, and Hades was following close behind him.

—*Revelation 6:8 (NIV)*

Chapter 8

THE ARMISTICE

For some, hope is sometimes a foreign idea in a city like early twentieth-century Butte. Most men worked incredibly long hours for low pay in dangerous conditions. Their wives and children never knew for certain if their men would return home, and a whistle from the mines at any time other than shift change usually meant that someone wouldn't. Hundreds of women made a dangerous and paltry living selling themselves in small shacks in back alleys. Sickness and accidental death were common. Labor unions incited violence that often turned against the very people the union wanted to protect. Hundreds of individuals and families made their homes in meager hovels on the side of a rocky hill, surrounded by smoggy, smoky air that often hid the beautiful mountains surrounding their valley. They scraped life from the rocks, praying every moment that the rocks wouldn't bury them.

For some, though, Butte was a second chance. The inhospitable, smoke-covered hill saved at least as many as it killed. It was an escape from famine, from war, or from abject poverty. "The Richest Hill on Earth" gave young men an opportunity to "make it." It gave them steady jobs to support their families. It gave a fortunate few young women the chance to have their own jobs and begin to support themselves away from the watchful eyes of parents, grandparents, and other relatives and neighbors who believed a young woman's main ambition should be that of wife and mother. As much as any American city in the early twentieth century, Butte offered young men and women the promise of some freedom and a bit of choice in the future.

By 1918, thousands of those who called Butte home had come from somewhere else. They came from other states, many of them from other mining towns in places like Michigan, Pennsylvania, Nevada, and Colorado. They came from the plains of Nebraska and South Dakota and from each coast—California and Connecticut. They journeyed from Minnesota, Missouri, Kentucky, Utah, Ohio, and New York. Just as many came from other corners of the world—Ireland and England, primarily, but also Austria, Germany, Finland, Italy, the Balkans, Mexico, and China. In 1918, about one-third of Butte's population had been born outside the United States. Of those who were native-born Americans, it was highly likely that at least one of their parents was not.

Butte, one historian writes, "was a microcosm of Europe," and in 1918, "Europe was at war."[101] While armies clashed on European battlefields, ethnic groups clashed in the streets of Butte. Recent German immigrants didn't want to fight against the Vaterland. Irishmen were wary of the American alliance with Britain. Socialists worried about what American intervention on the side of the Allies would do to their cause.[102] But if the Great War had fissured ethnic and racial relationships in Butte, the Armistice was the first step to healing them.

November began in Butte with a sense of hope. By the end of October, even though people were still dying, the Butte–Silver Bow Board of Health declared the epidemic "under controle [sic]."[103] Drs. Freund and Matthews grew cautiously optimistic. For the first week of November, the board members kept all previously ordered control measures in place. The emergency hospital remained open, arrangements were made with the Butte Police Department for officers to help ensure that crowds continued moving on the streets and sidewalks instead of stopping to gather, and the Columbia Bar was closed after it broke the infection control laws one too many times. The owner was arrested and fined, despite his protestations that the bartender was responsible for the violations. However, positive reports from the vaccine experiment at the county jail and hospital helped to further uplift the board's hopeful mood. The number of cases was declining, and "conditions looked more favorable" that the city had weathered the worst of the proverbial storm.[104]

Drs. Freund and Matthews had to feel that the longest month of their lives was finally coming to a close. On November 8, the board felt that "any further curtailment of business would be unnecessary....All Churches… and all places of Amusement…and all business of all kind" were allowed to resume as normal.[105] Dr. Freund was so pleased with the progress that he even advocated closing the temporary Red Cross hospital at Washington Middle School but was ultimately overruled. On November 11, the Butte–Silver Bow Board of Health agreed that "if the public used precausion [sic] there should be little worry" as the "Epedemic [sic] of Influenza had terminated."[106]

But triumph, not precaution, was the word of the day in Butte and around the nation on November 11, 1918. As news of the Armistice reached the city, her residents took to the streets in celebration. Thousands crowded Uptown Butte to march in parades, dance, drink, and sing patriotic songs. It's not hard to imagine a tired young miner standing in the middle of Montana Street on that seasonably chilly November evening. He attributed his fatigue to the long hours he'd worked recently, maybe some anxiety over not receiving a letter in several weeks from a brother or cousin who had been fighting overseas for quite some time. As church bells rang up and down the hill, though, he pushed the weariness aside and tried to ignore the aching in his bones. He and hundreds of others crowded in the street cheered. The chill he felt run up his spine and through his limbs was one, he thought, of patriotic emotion as he sang "When the Boys Come Home" as loudly as his sore throat would allow. Around him, strangers hugged and men pounded one another on the back. The miner decided to celebrate with a drink. Wiping sweat from his forehead despite the cool autumn air, he staggered into the saloon across the street, pushed his way to the bar, and shouted for a whiskey. The bartender shoved it across the counter and then waited impatiently, hand out. The miner dug in his pockets for coins. He held a handful up to his face, blew the dust off them, handed a couple over to the tender and drained the glass in a few quick swallows. The saloon was growing more crowded by the minute, and the roar of hundreds of excited men made his head pound. He pushed his empty glass across the bar, and the bartender quickly scooped it up, gave it a quick rinse, and immediately poured more whiskey into it for another thirsty patron. The young man made his way slowly through the throng of men and out into the Butte air. He was dizzy now; he probably drank the whiskey too fast, he thought. Within a few short days, he was dead. Cause of death: influenza and pneumonia.

Diseases rely on transmission from host to host. Without new, vulnerable hosts, the disease-causing microbe is unable to reproduce, eventually dying out in that particular area. Each infectious disease, though, has a different contagion level. This level is the disease's reproduction number, called an R_0 (pronounced "R naught"). The R_0 is calculated through accounting for the disease's contagious period, mode of transmission, and contact

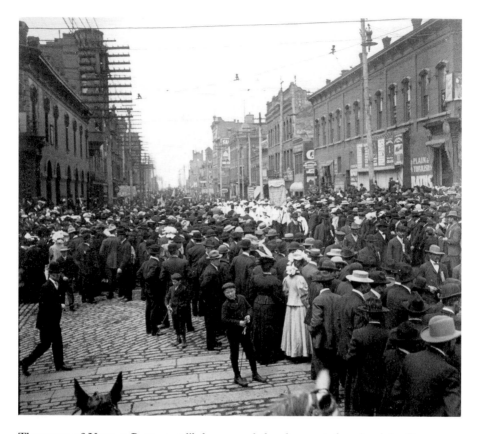

The streets of Uptown Butte were likely as crowded and congested on Armistice Day as they were on this circa 1915 Miners' Union Day celebration. *Montana Historical Society.*

rate—how many people an infected person is likely to come into contact with. Diseases with longer contagious periods have higher R_0s than those with shorter ones. Diseases that can spread through the air, like influenza, typically have higher R_0s than those that spread through blood or body fluids. Contact rate, though, can vary by geographic region due to cultural norms, public health practices, and healthcare systems. Thus, the specific R_0 varies not only from microbe to microbe but outbreak to outbreak. Researchers have calculated baseline R_0s for various common diseases, though. Measles, for example, is one the most contagious common viruses and has an estimated R_0 of 18. This means that a person infected with measles will pass the disease to, on average, 18 others. Comparatively, someone with seasonal influenza is likely to infect 1 other person. Seasonal flu has an R_0 of approximately 1.3, ranging from 0.9 to 2.1 depending on the season and strain. R_0s less than 1 indicate that an infection will die out, while R_0s greater than 1 have the potential to spread into the population, the extent growing ever-larger as the R_0 increases.[107]

The 1918 pandemic strain had an R_0 of approximately 2, ranging from 1.4 to 2.8. The exact R_0 depended on a variety of factors—population of a given area, living conditions, public health and healthcare systems, infrastructure, and the population's natural immunity to the virus. In isolated tribal communities on Native American reservations and in the Arctic and in the Pacific Islands, the R_0 and, consequently, the mortality rates were much higher than in the cities of the eastern United States. People in the cities were less likely to be part of a naïve population—a population that has no immunity to a disease because it's never experienced it or a related contagion. City dwellers were more likely to have access to healthcare and to be under the jurisdiction of an active and well-established public health system, though in some city neighborhoods, poor living conditions may have outweighed these benefits.

Accurately calculating the R_0 of a disease in a given area is a difficult task, especially when the outbreak is a century in the past. Without the ability to interview patients and track contacts, it's nearly impossible to calculate Butte's exact R_0 in 1918. It may have been higher or lower than for other areas, depending on all the extenuating circumstances. The Armistice celebration miner is hypothetical, but it's not a stretch to imagine a situation playing out in that manner. If such a situation followed the 1918 pandemic average and the miner infected two other Butte residents, it's easy to see how the disease exploded in the days following the celebration. The two people the miner infected passed the disease to four others, who, in turn, infected two each, creating eight cases. Those eight individuals each infected two people. The sixteen newly infected passed it to two each as well.

Spanish influenza's R_0 may pale in comparison to that of measles or mumps ($R_0 \sim 10$), but the increased suffering in Butte following Armistice Day defied statistics. On November 10, the day before the parades and celebrations, authorities reported only eight cases of influenza in the city. By November 12, that number had jumped to forty-four; ninety-two cases were reported on November 14, an elevenfold increase over the numbers the board had celebrated just a week earlier.[108] Influenza hadn't disappeared from Butte by November 11—it had simply been resting for a few days, and the very public, crowded, joyous Armistice Day celebrations gave it a longer leash on life, setting off a deadly chain of infection that burned through the city.

Chapter 9

THE PEOPLE VERSUS PUBLIC HEALTH

I f the first days of November brought the Butte–Silver Bow Board of Health hope, that feeling was gone by the month's second week. On November 14, Dr. Freund predicted "further increase in the numver [*sic*] of new cases within 24 hours," mainly due to the "recent Celebration."[109] Butte's public health officials were split on what actions to take. Some hesitated to reinstate stringent control measures, especially after the relative freedom Butte's residents had enjoyed in recent days. The increase in cases, however, was proof to others that the restriction-free movements had spread the illness to an extent beyond what they'd previously experienced. The board's first action was to order that all houses with influenza cases should be quarantined and placarded so that all passersby and potential visitors knew that the deadly disease was present in that home.

Today, as in 1918, public health officials have the legal authority to determine what measures should be put into place in order to stop the spread of communicable disease. Montana Code Annotated states that local boards of health have the authority and responsibility to "identify, assess, prevent, and ameliorate conditions of public health importance." This includes responsibilities for "epidemiological tracking and investigation" and "isolation and quarantine measures."[110] The wording isn't any more specific. In fact, local boards of health are given a lot of leeway to determine how to best control communicable diseases in their own jurisdictions. Local boards have the authority to "adopt regulations that do not conflict with rules adopted by the department" in order to control communicable disease.[111] In other words, local public health officials may develop their jurisdiction's own disease control regulations as long as they are not less stringent than those in state law. The Administrative Rules of Montana state, "If a communicable disease requires quarantine of contacts, a local health officer or the department shall institute whatever quarantine measures are necessary to prevent transmission."[112] The local health officer, with the approval of the local board of health, may determine the length, place, and other circumstances of quarantine as he or she deems necessary. The same is true for isolating infected patients.

Though some use the terms interchangeably, *isolation* and *quarantine* are different control measures for use in different circumstances. Isolation is reserved for persons infected with a communicable disease. The local board of health may determine that it is necessary to separate the infected person from others during the period of communicability to avoid the spread of infection. Alternately, quarantine is reserved for those who are not known to be infected but are at risk of contracting or spreading a disease because they have had or are in contact with someone who is known to be infected. Quarantine is most commonly utilized for household contacts, such as family members, of people infected with a communicable disease.

Since isolation and quarantine are among the most stringent of control measures, enforcing them comes with a great deal of responsibility on the part of the officials ordering them. One of the primary responsibilities is ensuring necessity. Since isolation and quarantine may be seen as a deprivation of certain civil liberties, the reasons for instigating those measures must be based on sound reasoning. Public health officials consider infection rates, incubation periods, modes of transmission, and the mortality rate of the pathogen in question. In Butte in 1918, the Butte–Silver Bow Board of Health was in unanimous agreement that the morbidity and mortality rates the city was experiencing made both isolation and quarantine measures necessary to protect the public's health. However, it also fully understood that the community would fight these. If they weren't ill, citizens would argue with directives to stay within their homes. People needed to go to work, to visit the grocer, to see their friends and family. They did not want the government dictating what they could and could not do any more than the American public would today. One can imagine that this feeling of independence was especially high in the triumphant days of patriotism following the Armistice.

Today, public health officials may begin this process by issuing voluntary quarantine orders. They reason that people may be more apt to comply

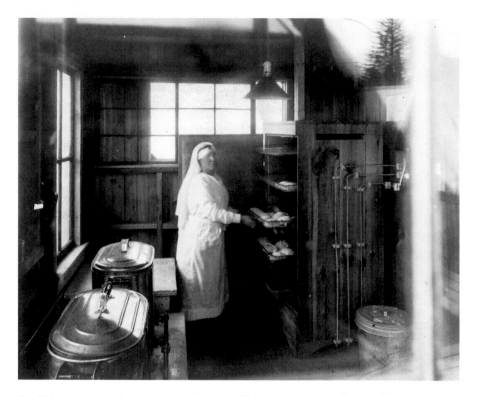

Sterilizing room, war influenza camp, Emery Hill, Lawrence, Massachusetts. *National Archives.*

with orders if they feel they have some autonomy and choice in the matter. Additionally, voluntary orders are less taxing on resources and come with fewer legal responsibilities. Once a local board of health issues mandatory isolation or quarantine orders, it takes responsibility for the issuees' basic needs—shelter, food, water, and even clothing, if necessary. The Butte–Silver Bow Board of Health, however, bypassed voluntary orders, instead moving directly to ordering formal mandatory quarantine for household contacts of influenza cases. Anyone who shared living quarters with someone infected with influenza was required to stay home, neither coming nor going for any reason. However, enforcing quarantine on that many people—hundreds, certainly, by mid- to late November—was a daunting task. To help carry it out, the board hired six "contagious guards…to inforce [*sic*] the Quarantine on all residence and places where the Influenza exist."[113] These men were paid $125 per month (almost $1,900 per month in today's money) to serve as sentinels, roaming the city to ensure that no one entered or left quarantined homes. Officials believed that if infection could be kept off the streets and inside individual homes, it would run out of hosts and eventually burn out.

Upon issuing mandatory isolation or quarantine orders, public health officials must ensure that the basic needs of the people under the orders are met and that they have access to any services they require. This may mean that public health workers take groceries to isolated or quarantined individuals, plus run their essential errands and arrange for visits from healthcare workers, members of the clergy, or other essential persons. The Butte–Silver Bow Board of Health enlisted the National Guard's assistance for these tasks. The National Guardsmen assisted the "contagious guards" enforcing quarantine by detaining violators and helping obtain food, medicine, and other things for the quarantined individuals. The men were given orders to "arrest any one violating such Quarantine, also, if any Person or persons under quarantine needed Medacine [sic] or Food, that it was the duty of the men on guard to purchase such."[114] Assuming that each person infected with influenza lived with at least one other, the number of people in Butte required to stay within their homes would have been about 250 on the day the quarantine order went into effect (127 cases were reported on November 22). In all actuality, the number was probably much higher. Many people had families—a spouse, children, parents, or grandparents—who lived with them. Many single miners lived in boardinghouses with several other men who, technically, were part of the quarantine order, though these were undoubtedly much more difficult to enforce. The number of people required to be under isolation or quarantine was simply too large for the city's few public health workers to care for themselves.[115]

Members of the public were not the only ones to voice their disagreement with the board of health's isolation and quarantine orders. Some of the city's physicians also disagreed with the measures. It wasn't that isolation and quarantine were completely unwarranted; the issue was more that the measures were entirely reactive and too little, too late. "The epidemic situation," members of the Silver Bow Medical Society stated, "demands sweeping measures."[116]

The Silver Bow Medical Society, which represented Butte's physicians, was led by Dr. Caroline McGill, who was no novice when dealing with contagious respiratory illness. Dr. McGill had first arrived in Butte on December 31, 1910. The first woman to earn a PhD from the University of Missouri, she'd come to the city to work as a pathologist at Murray Hospital. Far and away the most common things Dr. McGill identified in her lab each day were the rod-shaped bacteria of tuberculosis. "Consumption"

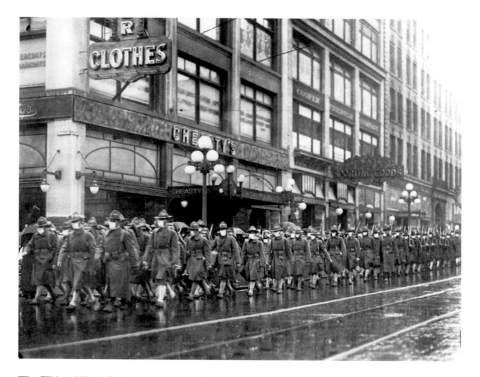

The Thirty-Ninth Regiment marched through the streets of Seattle, Washington, on its way to France. Everyone was provided with a mask made by the Seattle chapter of the Red Cross. *National Archives.*

was unfortunately common in Butte—the city was responsible for half of Montana's tuberculosis deaths in 1910—and fighting it became Dr. McGill's passion. She joined the Butte Anti-Tuberculosis Society and was instrumental in convincing the state legislature to fund a tuberculosis sanitarium. However, McGill believed that there was more she could do. She left Butte for two years to complete her medical degree at Johns Hopkins University, finishing at the top of her class.[117]

Back in Butte, Dr. McGill immediately returned to work serving the city's residents. She still treated Butte's many tuberculosis cases, but she also delivered babies, tended injuries obtained in the mines, and made house calls to the widows and children of men killed in the Granite Mountain–Speculator Disaster of 1917. She visited the city's saloons to tend to the injured after bar fights, and she called on the prostitutes in the Red Light District. She was highly intelligent, energetic, and compassionate.

She also spoke her mind. As president of the Silver Bow Medical Society, Dr. McGill led the group's "considerable criticism…at the health authorities for what was considered by some as laxity."[118] Isolation and quarantine are usually the last measures public health professionals choose to put in place in order to control disease. Instituting them in the absence of many other control measures, the society argued, was terribly inadequate and irresponsible. They believed the disease's incubation period needed to be factored in as well. People infected with influenza may not develop symptoms for up to four days but can spread the virus to others beginning a full day before the initial signs—fatigue, headache, and fever—set in. It was entirely probable that there were people walking the streets of Butte who were infected with influenza, were actively transmitting it to others, and had no idea. The Silver Bow Medical Society unanimously passed a number of resolutions aimed at encouraging, if not pressuring, the Butte–Silver Bow Board of Health to immediately enforce "vigorous and stringent measures," including closing all businesses "not essential to life," prohibiting public gatherings and keeping schools closed.[119] In short, Dr. McGill and the Silver Bow Medical Society heartily recommended that Butte return to its pre-Armistice state—quiet, motionless, and isolated. It was the only way to stem the tide of infection.

Public health works at a community-wide level, basing decisions on what is best for the community as a whole. The physician's perspective, however, is generally based on the individual patient, sometimes widening to those in closest proximity to the patient. The doctors on and working with the Butte–Silver Bow Board of Health had a clear understanding of both perspectives. They knew that the return of stringent control measures and community-wide closures would help slow or stop the spread of infection. However, they also understood that a massive amount of public opposition would come their way. Their predicament is far from enviable. The Silver Bow Medical Society's resolutions effectively tasked board members with weighing the financial, ethical, and civic costs of a complete citywide activity ban with the potential benefit to the health of the public at-large.

Dr. Freund, the only board of health member who also belonged to the Silver Bow Medical Society, agreed with McGill and his fellow society colleagues. His decision is notable. As secretary of the board of health, Freund was tasked with much of the groundwork for ensuring its resolutions and measures were followed. Adopting the medical society's resolutions would almost certainly create greater strain for the board of health and himself. His agreement illustrates his ardent belief that such measures were necessary.

Still, the board of health balked. A representative of the United States Medical Corps posted in Butte had previously advised board members that such widespread closures would not be necessary. Rather, the strict quarantine should help to prevent any further cases. Closures would only stop influenza as long as businesses and organizations stayed closed. Once they reopened, "the Influenza would again increase."[120] So instead of full business closures, the board initially added softer measures, like prohibiting bargain sales in stores and not closing but limiting congestion in saloons.

The board of health also chose, in addition to continuing quarantine efforts, to focus on sanitation. Dr. Freund was tasked with meeting with laundry owners "to discuss the best means for handling laundry in a sanitary manner."[121] An inspection of the city's boardinghouses was ordered. Home and business owners were no longer allowed to sweep their sidewalks unless they used "a Compound as a dust preventative." Additionally, "the streets would be flushed when necessary to prevent unnecessary dust."[122] It was entirely possible, board members reasoned, that the contagion was carried in the air, so it must certainly latch itself to dust particles. Avoid dust swirling through the air and avoid the influenza it carried. This belief hearkens back to the days of miasma theory, showing just how much this virulent, terrible influenza made these practiced doctors and professionals doubt and question their years of training and experience.

Still, the numbers showed no improvement: 586 total cases in the week ending on November 23; 15 deaths on November 22; 19 on the twenty-fourth; 9 on the twenty-sixth; 13 on the twenty-seventh. Saddled with these increasing morbidity and mortality rates and faced with continued pressure from Drs. Freund and McGill, the board of health finally concurred with the Silver Bow Medical Society's suggestions. On November 29, with Dr. McGill and other medical society members in attendance, the Butte–Silver Bow Board of Health officially passed the following resolution:

> *WHEREAS, it appears at the present time to the Silver Bow County Medical Society, there is an epidemic of Influenza, and*
> *WHEREAS, it appears to the County Board of Health of Silver Bow County, Montana, that the epidemic of influenza is again rapidly increasing, and*
> *WHEREAS, it is further made to appear to said County Board of Health that one of the causes of the spreading of said disease is a congregation of people in public spaces and upon public streets and highways.*
> *THEREFORE, BE IT RESOLVED, that all places of business and amusement, including Churches and schools be, and the same are hereby ordered closed; excepting however, food supply stores, restaurants and boarding houses.*

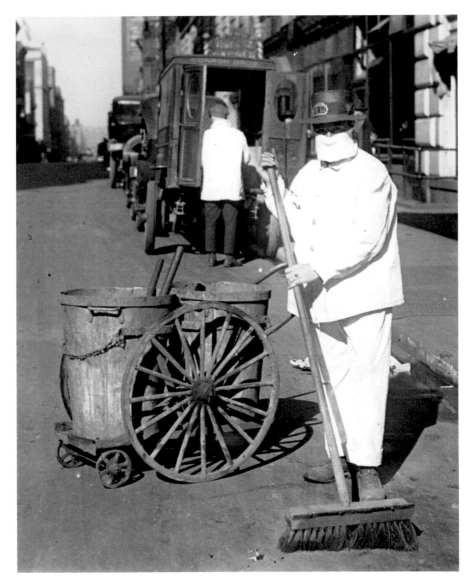

In a scene repeated around the country, street cleaners in New York City wear masks as they clean the streets. One official reportedly said of the masks, "Better ridiculous than dead." *National Archives.*

BE IT FURTHER RESOLVED, that clothing stores be opened only for the purpose of supplying absolute necessities; that drug stores be opened only for the purpose of supplying necessities and filling prescriptions.
BE IT FURTHER RESOLVED, that all clerks, waiters, waitresses and other waiting on the public be compelled to wear masks.
BE IT FURTHER RESOLVED, that at no time shall any number of people congregate on the public streets and highways of the City of Butte, and upon the public roads and highways of Silver Bow County; and the Sheriff of Silver Bow County and the Chief of Police of the City of Butte, are hereby directed to stringently enforce this resolution.[123]

Copies of the resolution were distributed to the mayor, police chief, sheriff, and "Sanitary Inspectors," and it went into full effect promptly at 8:00 a.m. the next day.[124]

Once again, usually bustling Butte came to a standstill. Shops closed, theaters remained dark, and the roller coaster at Columbia Gardens stood motionless. The National Guardsmen assisting with quarantines were given the additional task of ensuring that crowds in the streets didn't get too large. Once a group started to form, the Guardsmen were under order to break it up and encourage people to move along. The board of health couldn't very well quarantine the population of an entire city, but Dr. Freund and the others hoped that keeping the contact Butte's residents had with one another to an absolute minimum would help keep the transmission rate low.

Unsurprisingly, the people of Butte pushed back. "When a burglar is caught, the authorities do not lock up the public to make them safe from the burglar—they lock up the burglar," a theater advertisement stated. "Why not quarantine the 'flu' and let the well folks go about their business????" the ad continued. The theater owners added some statistics of their own to bolster the argument: "Approximately one hundred theatergoers and not one of them has the flu…Epidemic? Well, we have our own little private opinion based on figures and not on what someone thinks."[125] The theater's advertisement did more than disagree with the strict measures. It illustrated the distrust that many in Butte felt toward their authorities. Perhaps those who had ill friends or family members understood the seriousness of the disease, but it may still have been difficult for them, and especially those untouched by influenza, to understand the necessity of essentially shutting down public life. Were these measures really about public safety, people wondered, or were they about public control?

Business owners were especially incensed about the order. After all, their livelihoods depended on customers and regular business hours. A number of them presented the board of health with alternate solutions to the complete shutdown. They suggested that instead of complete closure, they only allow a certain number of patrons in at a time. The entrepreneurs pledged to forego advertisements that would entice more customers in or accept returns or exchanges of goods. They even offered to pay a public health official to stay within their business during open hours to ensure none of the new enforcements were breached. The board of health took the suggestions "under advisement" but left the original resolution in place—essentially a "thanks, but no thanks" answer to the suggestions.[126] If any of the restrictions were modified or lifted too soon, public health officials would never truly know how successful they had been. It's also possible the board believed that if exceptions were made for certain types of business, other businesses and organizations would expect the same. Once put into place, the strict quarantine would remain in effect until case numbers, not public approval or disapproval, warranted its lifting.

Miscommunication between agencies contributed to public discontent. Toward the end of the month, the board of health fielded several complaints about local businesses failing to comply with closures and restrictions. The Butte police, it seems, told several business owners that compliance with the public health orders was voluntary. The board members cleared up this misunderstanding quickly, even threatening to call on Montana's governor to supply troops to enforce the measures within the city. One can imagine the outrage business owners must have felt upon receiving two different sets of instructions, both from public authorities, within such a short amount of time.[127]

The board of health had one final order. As a last precaution, any victim of influenza or pneumonia was to be placed in a closed casket with his or her face and head wrapped within twenty-four hours of death.[128] Any infractions of this measure were considered misdemeanors. Stopping influenza became a matter of controlling not just the living but also the dead. And there were many of them. Influenza took over three hundred from Butte in November 1918—a greater toll than it ever had taken before or has taken since.[129]

Chapter 10

TRAGIC IRONY

Visnes, Norway, on the country's west coast and located about one hundred miles south of Bergen, was home to one of Europe's largest copper mines in the late nineteenth century. Christian Visnes was born here in 1885. His family may not have been copper miners, but Christian, along with his wife, Magdalene, certainly understood the ins and outs of life in a copper mining town. They decided to try their luck in America, where Christian could practice his home village's trade in the world's largest copper-producing city: Butte. The journey from Norway took the couple through Liverpool and Boston before they finally arrived in Montana. By the fall of 1918, the Visneses had made a comfortable life for themselves in Butte. Christian worked in the mines, and Magdalene tended their home and two-year-old son Norman in Central Butte, just a block over from Christian's bachelor brother John.[130]

Christian was the first of the family to fall that fateful November in Butte. He died on the seventh of influenza and "lung congestion." Magdalene took ill the next day. Grieving and possibly too ill to care for herself or her son, she and Norman moved into her brother-in-law John's home. Magdalene probably didn't make it to her husband's November 10 burial. Instead, she was almost certainly in bed, coughing uncontrollably and shivering with fever, her lips and extremities slowly turning blue from lack of oxygen. She died the next day and was buried next to Christian in Butte's Mount Moriah Cemetery. Neither reached the age of thirty-five. Norman, too young to remember either of his parents, was raised by his uncle.[131]

Christian and Magdalene Visnes illustrate one of the most disturbing and unique characteristics of the 1918–19 influenza virus: its preference for young, otherwise healthy adults. Influenza, both seasonal and pandemic strains, most often targets the very young and very old, creating a U-shaped mortality curve. Excess deaths occur at each end of the life span but taper off in between. The 1918 strain did kill the young and old, but quite unusually, adults between the ages of twenty and forty years old accounted for nearly half the deaths in the United States. The average age of influenza victims in 1918 was thirty-three—Christian Visnes's age at death.

Epidemiologists did not chart the 1918 pandemic's mortality patterns on the usual U-shaped curve. Instead, the plotted line is more the shape of an upside-down V—opposite the usual curve—with excess mortality dropping significantly among the elderly.[132] This peculiarity made Butte especially susceptible. In 1918, over 50 percent of the city's residents were between the ages of twenty and forty-four. Thus, the majority of Butte's residents were vulnerable to influenza simply because of their age. This age group (twenty to forty-four) accounted for over 70 percent of Butte's pandemic victims. The virus took an extreme toll on Butte's young adults disproportionate to the rest of the city's residents.[133]

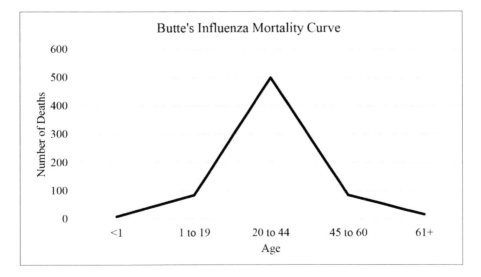

A mortality curve illustrates the mortality rate of a disease epidemic. Influenza mortality curves are usually U-shaped, with mortality highest in young children and older adults. The 1918 pandemic mortality curve was opposite. *Author's collection.*

There are several explanations for this unique mortality curve. Recent scientific research puts some of the blame on the immune system itself. Researchers theorize that the old and young died when the virus overwhelmed their naturally weak immune systems. In some young adults, though, the disease was unable to overpower strong immune systems. Instead, influenza manipulated the immune system into overreacting to the virus, resulting in a condition now referred to as Acute Respiratory Distress Syndrome (ARDS). This condition is an immune response that works in a way similar to an allergic reaction. For example, if someone has an allergy to pollen, his or her immune system will immediately identify pollen as a dangerous invader and mount an aggressive response. The respiratory inflammation; itchy, watery eyes; and sneezing are all part of that response. In effect, it isn't the pollen that makes an allergy sufferer feel sick but the body's response to the invader.

This was sometimes the case with influenza. Upon infection, strong immune systems mounted an immediate and powerful attack on the virus. In some instances, as is possible in the case of Christian Visnes, the massive release of immune proteins sent to battle the virus ended up overwhelming the delicate structures that allow blood and oxygen to circulate through the lungs. Visnes would have struggled for breath as his lungs filled with blood, fluid, and other debris and ultimately stopped functioning. During an autopsy, the physician would find Visnes's lungs filled with fluid and blood. This explains how "lung congestion" was labeled as a contributing factor in Visnes's death. Like hundreds of other young adults in 1918 and 1919, Visnes drowned in his own immune response.

In other cases, ARDS caused organ failure due to lack of oxygen. Heart failure, for instance, occurred when the organ didn't have enough oxygen available to pump blood. Other victims died of exhaustion. They had to breathe so rapidly and work so hard for air that the lungs and other muscles simply gave out. In these cases, the body systems that usually saved young adults from the horrors of disease may have been what led to their deaths. In a disease experience that accounted for too many cruelties to count, this tragic irony is perhaps one of the most bitter.[134]

But Christian Visnes was doubly susceptible to influenza in 1918 due not only to age but sex as well. In the United States, the male death rate was 50 percent higher than the female rate, a statistic that held true in Butte as well, even when taking into account that the population was majority male (almost 6,000 more men lived in Butte than women). If mortality rates between the sexes were even, one might expect approximately 245 influenza deaths in males in Butte. Instead, the actual number was more than twice that. The reasons for the high male death rate, though, are only speculative. Young men were less likely to stay home and rest when ill, possibly allowing the disease to progress beyond the point of treatment. Men generally also spent more time outside the home than women. Christian Visnes, for instance, left home to work in the mines each day, in close quarters with other men. Time spent outside the home led to more contact with new microbes, which may have had one of two negative effects: strengthening immune systems, increasing the chances of developing ARDS; or weakening immune systems, creating vulnerability to stronger bacteria and viruses, like the 1918 strain of influenza. Or the reason for the male mortality rate may be a combination of these or other factors.

BUTTE INFLUENZA DEATHS BY GENDER

Data Set	Male	Female
Total Population	22,314	16,851
Influenza Deaths	517	189
Percentage	2.3 percent	1.1 percent

What is apparent from these examples is that influenza in 1918 may not have purposefully discriminated, but it had preferences. The virus's primary goals were survival and reproduction, and it found its best chances for those in young, healthy men. The exact reasons why are still unknown. Influenza, after all, "is, by its very nature, fundamentally unpredictable."[135]

Chapter 11

INEQUALITY IN DEATH

C hristian and Magdalene Visnes were only two of over three hundred deaths directly caused by influenza and pneumonia recorded in Butte in November. The Metz family also found itself among the number suffering with illness and loss that month. John and Louisa Metz came to Butte from Germany before the turn of the twentieth century. They worked a small farm near Tivoli Brewery on Butte's western outskirts where they raised four sons: Henry, twenty-eight; Fred, twenty-five; Dan, thirteen; and Arthur, eleven. Fred's wife, Nellie, twenty-five, also lived on the farm, where she helped with household chores and cared for the couple's one-year-old daughter, Helen Jean. Influenza struck the family in late November. The number of family members who fell ill is unknown, but Nellie and her brother-in-law Henry were the Metzes' first casualties. Instead of trying to fight the disease at home like many did, family members took them to St. James Hospital. The family may have hoped that with hospital care, Nellie and Henry could recover more quickly. The comfort and care available at the hospital was, they perhaps believed, superior to what they could provide on the farm. It's also possible that the family took the two to the hospital as a kind of self-instituted isolation and quarantine. Removing the two sick persons from the house would, hopefully, help ensure that the rest of the family remained safe from the illness. However well-thought out and intentioned the reason, the efforts were futile. Fred fell ill shortly after

Henry and Nellie were moved to St. James. Henry and Nellie both died at the hospital on November 24, and Fred succumbed to influenza at the family's home that same day. Helen Jean became one of the hundreds of Butte's newly orphaned that autumn and winter. Unlike so many, though, she was fortunate enough to have relatives to care for her.[136]

The Metz family's tragedy offers some important clues and insights into the behavior of the influenza virus circulating in Butte and the rest of the nation in 1918. John and Louisa Metz were both over the age of fifty in 1918. Their age placed them in a group that was usually especially susceptible to influenza, but as the cases of their sons and daughter-in-law illustrate, this wasn't the 1918 strain's usual preference. Perhaps it was their age that saved them. However, their survival may also be attributed to another factor—the time at which they had immigrated.

Despite the turmoil and confusion it brought to Butte and communities worldwide in 1918, influenza was not a new disease. Pandemic influenza had struck as recently as 1889–90, and just two years later, in 1892, an influenza epidemic ravaged America. Scientists later discovered the 1892 influenza strain was very genetically similar to the 1918 strain. Anyone who contracted influenza in 1892 should have had some immunity to infection in 1918. However, the 1892 epidemic was restricted to the United States. Later immigrants had no exposure to this strain so no chance to acquire even partial immunity to the 1918 strain. Perhaps this helps explain why John and Louisa, who had immigrated before 1892, survived while later immigrants, like Christian and Magdalene Visnes, died. The Metzes had immigrated in time to possibly come in contact with the 1892 strain, thereby gaining some immunity to the 1918 strain. However, their sons and daughter-in-law, the Visneses, and hundreds of others in Butte were either born or immigrated later than 1892.[137]

All over the United States, immigrants had a higher pandemic mortality rate than native-born Americans. In Butte, the issues of ethnicity and immigration were amplified. Over 30 percent of the city's population was foreign-born (in comparison, approximately 24 percent of all Montanans were immigrants), and a large proportion of Butte's immigrants fit into the twenty-to-forty-four age bracket, products of the early twentieth-century immigration rush. In fact, 70 percent of Butte's immigrants were between the ages of twenty and forty-four, making them doubly susceptible to influenza in 1918. Though native-born Americans outnumbered immigrants in Butte by more than two to one, influenza killed both populations in nearly equal numbers in 1918.[138]

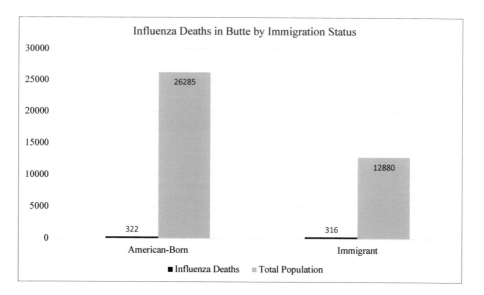

The immigrant mortality rate was 2.4 percent, while the mortality rate for American-born residents was half that at 1.2 percent. *Author's collection.*

The argument over immigration is an old one, with discrimination against various groups changing to meet the social issues and economic demands of the time. In the early twentieth century, especially in the era of World War I, many people in Butte despised the "bohunks," the city's Balkan immigrants. They accused "these black men from across the water" of stealing jobs that should have gone to "white men."[139] In later years, the Balkan immigrants who weathered the prejudice and stayed in Butte became some of the city's most respected citizens. Spiro Vucinich, age forty-four, was among Butte's earlier Balkan immigrants. Born in Serbia, he had lived in Butte for nineteen years and was naturalized in 1902. Spiro was a well-known merchant, a partner in the firm of Vucinich & Angelich.[140] He and his younger wife, Soka, twenty-eight—also a Balkan immigrant—had four children. In mid-November, their youngest son, one-year-old Veleko, fell ill with influenza. Spiro and Soka were helpless as their boy grew weaker and struggled for breath. He died on November 21. The parents barely had time to mourn before the disease struck both of them as well. Less than one week later, they were also dead. They left behind three other children.[141]

Clementina Marianetti from Italy, Pablo Zarragoitia of Spain, Austrian-born housewife Gertrude Sithes, Swedish American ranch hand Emil Sjoguist, and Edward O'Rourke of Ireland were among the dozens of names from each of Butte's ethnic communities appearing in the death records of 1918 with a listed cause of influenza and pneumonia. As fall turned to winter in 1918, influenza continued its deadly sweep through the city. Though the rest of the year proved less deadly than November, the deaths continued, and more disturbing patterns illustrating influenza's preferences slowly became apparent.[142]

PART IV

DECEMBER 1918

Now is the winter of our discontent.

—*William Shakespeare,* Richard III

Chapter 12

THE UNFORTUNATE AND THE FORGOTTEN

December 1918 dawned quiet, cold, and still in Butte. The winter sun rose slowly over the eastern ridge as if frozen in the icy air. Shrouded in fog and smoke from the smelter fires, its bright rays shone dully on the city, letting out little heat. The people of Butte shrank even further into their homes, huddling in corners and near stoves, wrapped in blankets to ward off the winter chill and the threat of illness. Every cough and sniffle, usually so commonplace and unconcerning in the coldest months of the Rocky Mountain winter, was now viewed with fear and suspicion. Did the children shiver from the chill, or was it the beginnings of the deadly fever? Was the miner coughing to clear the underground dust from his lungs, or had he been infected with influenza?

As they watched medical professionals struggle to help their dying family members, friends, and neighbors, the people of Butte increasingly turned not only to patent medicines but also their own folk remedies to help treat influenza. They hung camphor and garlic around their necks, gargled disinfectants, and took steam baths. They made chest poultices of clay, turpentine, and mustard and medicated themselves with whiskey, opium, and strychnine. These home treatments provided no real relief and did nothing to stop the spread of the flu.[143]

There was one folk remedy in Butte, though, that claimed some success, and it came from Chinatown. Butte's Chinatown was an area of about two square blocks, roughly bounded by Main, Silver, Colorado, and Galena Streets, and it was here that Dr. Huie Pock, an "acupuncturist, herbalist, and surgeon," practiced Eastern medicine for almost fifty years. He didn't just treat the city's Chinese residents; his remedies were quite popular with a number of Butte inhabitants, despite the fact that he practiced without a medical license. He offered to test for one, "but there was no test for Chinese medicine, thus he had no license."[144] Despite his popularity, Dr. Pock's practice wasn't scandal-free. He occasionally was called to defend himself against multiple malpractice charges, sometimes successfully, sometimes not.[145]

If the reports can be believed, Dr. Pock seemed to have a successful treatment for influenza. The doctor reportedly packed salt behind the patient's knees and in the armpits. This, allegedly, drew the "toxins" to those areas, where they could be removed by syringe. Various natural health advocates over the years have touted the healing value of salt, and there is some evidence that it may help reduce inflammation and draw out infection, especially from open wounds. However, it's highly unlikely that Dr. Pock's treatment cured influenza, as suggested by the *Butte Miner*—"Heathen Chinese Has a Flu Cure," a headline announced on November 30, 1918. The remedy may have had a placebo effect or provided relief for some of influenza's symptoms, and an unknown number of Butte's residents ventured to Chinatown to attempt the "cure," but it's impossible to know how many of them it may have helped, if any at all.[146]

Despite Dr. Pock's popularity and success both in and out of Chinatown, most of the neighborhood's residents lived anonymous lives within its borders. Even into the twentieth century, the Chinese were undercounted in censuses and, if counted at all, often not recorded by name. Instead, census records sometimes show "a name spelled forward and backward and finally crossed out with the word 'Chinaman' written in over the scratched lines."[147] The Chinese were disparaged due to their strange dress, their proclivity for wearing their hair in long braids, and their language. Even in a city where a number of different languages were spoken on the streets, the Chinese language was an anomaly, strange to both the eyes and ears of Butte's largely Anglo-European population. The Chinese residents' food preferences—rice, vegetables, and fish as opposed to red meats, bread, and beans—were odd, and their use of opium, though liberally used in patent medicines, was considered immoral. Polite society viewed the opium dens as the haunts of prostitutes and unemployed drunks. In Chinatown's alleys and back rooms, opium was not a medicine but a vice. The city that was a "microcosm of Europe" had no room for a piece of East Asia.[148]

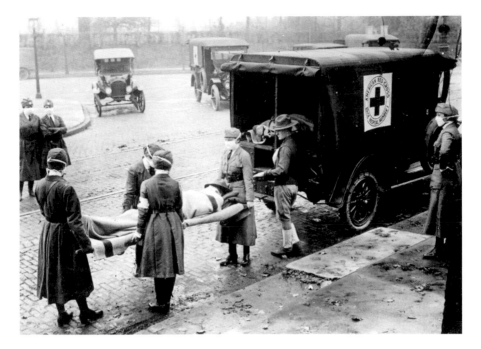

St. Louis, Missouri, Red Cross Motor Corps on duty. *National Archives.*

The Chinese weren't alone in their isolation in Butte. The city's Red Light District sat next to the shops, noodle parlors, and opium dens of Chinatown. Both neighborhoods were roughly the same size. The Red Light District lay within the approximate borders of Main, Park, Arizona, and Mercury Streets. Many of its brothels were large high-class houses, with luxurious drapes and furniture, run by wealthy madams. The women who lived and worked within them, especially on the main floors, were well dressed and carefully groomed. They entertained men at large parties and then privately in their own fashionably furnished rooms. A number of smaller, less extravagant rooms lined the hallways of the houses' basements, with a woman living and working in each one.

The alleys just behind the great, warm, well-lit brothel houses were a maze of makeshift shacks made of scraps of tin and rough boards. The majority of the district's women spent their short, dangerous lives in these small "cribs," providing entertainment for the men either unable to afford the brothels' prices or unwelcome in those houses because of their propensity to cause trouble. All of the district's women, but especially those living in the alleyway cribs, lived under the constant threat of violence and poverty. Some of the women had been born into that life, part of a seemingly unbreakable cycle. Unemployment had forced others there. A few chose it for themselves. Many turned to opium or alcohol to help soothe their existence.

Due to its naturally secretive nature, records on life in the Red Light District are hard to find. City officials usually turned a blind eye to the district's business dealings, and this included neglecting to keep and maintain accurate counts and records of the women living there. By January 1917, most Americans believed the nation's entry into World War I was inevitable, and Butte officials finally cracked down on the district's business. As part of an effort to keep the city's potential soldiers healthy and free of sexually transmitted infections, Butte's "working women" were forced out of town or arrested. By the fall of 1918, it's possible that some had returned or a new group of unfortunates had moved in to continue the business, but the district was never as large or busy as it had been before the closure.

In a city made of various ethnic and class-stratified neighborhoods, Chinatown and the Red Light District were the outliers—places that were often frequented by men and women from all levels of the city's socioeconomic spectrum but almost always in secret. Consequently, the residents of Chinatown and the Red Light District had a cordial and cooperative relationship. In the district's heyday, its women would visit Chinatown herbalists and doctors for their medical issues. If any women remaining in the district during the fall of 1918 contracted influenza, it's possible that they sought care from Chinese physicians like Dr. Pock.

Unfortunately, the district women's plight during this terrible time is as mysterious as that of the Chinese population. Butte's hundreds of "unseen" residents likely suffered morbidity and mortality rates at least as high, if not higher, as those officially recorded. The residents of the Red Light District were not in a position to take advantage of the nursing care Red Cross volunteers provided. Only the most charitable and compassionate of volunteers would be willing to visit the area, and even then in limited capacity. Most of the women of the district were poor and, especially if ill, would have had trouble tending to their own daily needs on their own— food, warmth, even decent shelter. Butte winters are bone-chillingly cold, and it's difficult to keep a tin shack in an alley warm.

Conversely, though, the severity of influenza may have helped keep Chinatown and the Red Light District relatively healthy. If isolation and quarantine orders and business closures kept the rest of Butte more separated than usual, it's possible that the already segregated communities of Chinatown and the Red Light District saw fewer visitors than normal, offering influenza fewer chances to spread. Without records, however, the pandemic experience of Butte's Chinese and Red Light District residents is unfortunately lost to history, just like so many other facets of their lives.

Chapter 13
SINNERS AND SAINTS

While the people of Butte did all they could to keep influenza out of their homes and from stealing their loved ones, the city's public health officials worked tirelessly to do the same. December began with a continuation of the battle over mandatory closures. Business owners weren't the only people testing the boundaries. Some of the city's doctors, in an effort to ease the hardships quarantine placed on the families they served, began purposefully misidentifying cases of influenza as pneumonia, thus allowing their patients' households to avoid quarantine. After visiting the patients in their homes, the physicians saw firsthand the hardship that quarantine placed on family members. Quarantined, but healthy, adults were unable to work, and families suffered financially. Those in quarantine were dependent on government officials to ensure they had adequate food and other supplies. Butte's doctors didn't see the misdiagnoses as negligent; after all, they were providing care to the ill. They simply had a very different perspective on the epidemic than did the members of the Butte–Silver Bow Board of Health. Most physicians didn't hear the case numbers each day—the total numbers of the ill and the dead—as the board members did. Instead, they visited some of those afflicted people in their homes and saw, firsthand, the devastation that the disease brought to its victims and the hardships that its effects bestowed on a patient's family members. Their experience was more than a collection of numbers but a collection of faces. Butte's physicians understood the seriousness of influenza just as well as public health officials, just in a very different way. Both groups had the same goal: to ease the city's suffering. However, where the board of health used community-wide control measures to contain the disease, many of the city's doctors saw the solution through providing care and meeting the needs of patients and household members on an individual basis. Each perspective and method was well intentioned, but in an environment as tense and wrought with worry as Butte in late 1918, there was no room left for alternative views. The board of health, with the power of government behind it, won the day, ordering that all cases of pneumonia needed to be reported and quarantined, effectively closing the loophole.[149]

Butte laid approximately fifty influenza victims to rest in the first week of December—half as many as the week prior. Though weary and still filled with fear, some in the city began to breathe gentle sighs of relief. The closures and quarantines had certainly helped, but after more than eight weeks of dealing with the scourge, most people had already contracted influenza and recovered or been fortunate enough to have immune systems that resisted infection. The disease, it seems, was finally beginning to run out of victims in Butte.

Health officials agreed. After threatening noncompliant businesses with military intervention just a little over a week earlier, by December 7, board members determined that businesses should be allowed to reopen. This directive included shops, restaurants, barbershops, saloons, and pool halls but with restrictions on crowd sizes and directives aimed at limiting the amount of time people spent in one place around other patrons. For instance, "no chairs [were to] be allowed in saloons" to avoid large crowds from forming. "Churches, theaters, dance halls, public gatherings, and places of amusement," though, were still under the closed order. In all other instances, the businesses' economic benefits once again outweighed the public health concern.[150]

Of course, Butte's religious leaders vehemently disagreed with the board of health's decision. Having their churches categorized as "places of amusement" undoubtedly rankled Butte's religious officials, and they took offense to the fact that saloons and pool halls should be allowed to operate while their places of worship could not. This battle, not necessarily between good and evil but between entities that some viewed as opposing ends of a moral spectrum, had begun in October when Reverend Chapman declared that "not only are all men equal before the law, but... all public dangers are equal before the law....Our institutions and national declarations stand for vital facts in the life of the people."[151] If churches could not hold service, church representatives argued, saloons should also close. The argument went much deeper, though, and hit to the core of what purposes both of these institutions served and what they meant to their neighborhoods and patrons.

For many in Butte, the neighborhood church was the center of the community. By 1918, the city boasted forty-seven churches, missions, and synagogues. These institutions baptized babies, educated children, performed marriages, and provided other social services to their members. The Catholic Church especially provided a sense of stability in transitory Butte. Almost half of the city's citizens belonged to a Catholic parish. Services in the church buildings themselves may have been banned, but there was nothing to stop priests from visiting private residences and performing rites in congregants' homes, and certainly many did. Influenza may have been life and death, but for many of Butte's people, their relationship with God meant eternity.[152]

Reverend Patrick Brosnan was one of the clergymen who continued visiting his parish members despite public health warnings and restrictions. Reverend Brosnan, twenty-six, left County Kerry, Ireland, in mid-1916, landing first at St. Thomas's Rectory in Cornwall-on-Hudson, New York, before receiving an appointment to St. Mary's Parish in Butte. It was, he wrote his father in February 1917 after his arrival, "a very good parish" with "five masses every Sunday and all of them crowded."[153]

As influenza spread through Butte, Reverend Brosnan made himself available day and night to tend to the sick and dying of his parish. "His zeal for the poor and lowly of the parish and city knew no bounds," the *Butte Miner* reported, "and he was ever at their command."[154] Reverend Brosnan's visits in the autumn of 1918 took him to countless residences where he prayed over the sick and performed rites for the dying. But the selfless care of his parishioners took a toll. He fell ill on October 31 and was advised to remain in bed. Instead, Reverend Brosnan continued to visit the needy members of St. Mary's until he died at St. James Hospital on November 10. "When reading the lives of the saints I have always thought that only their virtues were presented to us while their faults were obscured," wrote Brosnan's mentor, Father Michael Hannan. "In Father Brosnan I beheld a saint endowed with every saintly virtue and as free from faults and shortcomings as it is at all possible from our poor frail human nature to be."[155]

Butte, though, is a study in contrasts—"yesterday, today, and probably tomorrow she is a city of paradox."[156] Selfless service like Reverend Brosnan's was not confined to the city's religious communities. Most of Butte's residents depended on the semi-permanent mining industry, which

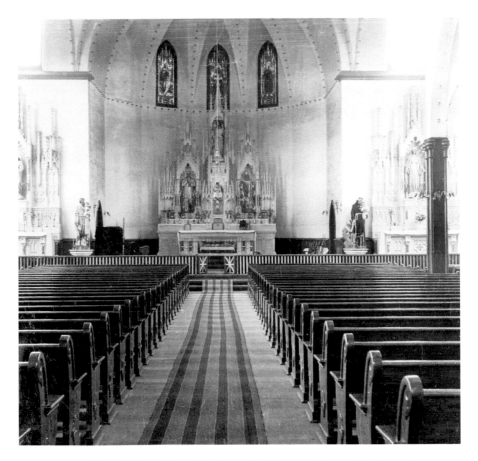

The interior of Sacred Heart Church before the building was damaged by fire and reconstructed in 1912. *Montana Historical Society.*

followed cyclical "boom and bust" periods. Men might stay in Butte for a few months or years and then follow the boom to other parts of the country—places like Michigan, Colorado, or Arizona—where their mining experience may help them finally make the fortune they hadn't quite been able to acquire in Butte. When that boom inevitably ended, some made their way back to Montana. Even if they returned to the same mines they'd worked in months or years before, the shafts and crosscuts were likely unfamiliar. New underground tunnels had been dug in their absence and staffed with men they didn't know. Creating a sense of community was difficult, and residents, especially the city's various ethnic populations, depended on neighborhood establishments—churches but also saloons and pool halls—to foster a sense of belonging. The same young Irish immigrant who took Mass at St. Patrick's on Sunday frequented his neighborhood pub each day after his shift. Saloonkeepers and pool hall owners, while businessmen, sometimes also filled the vital roles of community leaders in Butte neighborhoods.

In 1918, nearly one-quarter of Butte's population was Irish-born or the children of Irish immigrants, and Irish keepers ran almost 30 percent of the city's saloons. The city's German, Slavic, Italian, English, and Finnish communities all had their own saloons as well, each with a defining ethnic culture. Many of the city's saloons provided vital social services for the poor and those on the fringes, just as the churches did. They served as the neighborhoods' unofficial community halls, news outlets, and even banks. Due to language and cultural differences, many immigrants felt more comfortable visiting neighborhood saloons than official agencies for resources and assistance. Instead, they turned to places like Dublin Dan's "Hobo Retreat." Dublin Dan's, on the corner of Main and Porphyry, boasted a giant pot of stew, constantly simmering and available for anyone in need. Clotheslines ran along the back walls, and after the bar closed, men laid blankets on the floor to sleep. Closing saloons like Dublin Dan's disrupted more than after-work drinking. Many of the "regulars" had few other options for food, shelter, and company. Saloon proprietors' decision to ignore the order to close or change business practices is no surprise. On October 17 alone, twenty-three men were arrested for congregating in a closed pool hall, and a week later, saloon proprietor Thomas Connolly was arrested for "selling beer in glasses." No doubt the *Anaconda Standard*'s headline ("Saloonman Held for Selling Over a Bar") stirred up resentment for those measures. Such a harsh punishment, it suggested, for an innocuous act.[157] On November 4 and 5, two more saloons were closed for violating orders.

The untold stories behind these infractions, though, may go much deeper than men simply pining for their after-shift drink. The pool hall, Connolly's establishment, and the two saloons closed in early November may have served as home, even if only for a night or two, to men jumping from boardinghouse to boardinghouse or those who were never promised a regular bed wherever they usually paid their rent. Miners, railroad workers, and others without permanent shelter depended on hotels, rooming houses, and, in some cases, the saloons and pool halls in their respective ethnic neighborhoods.[158]

The story of one man in Butte illustrates the deep need the city, like all others, had for services. On November 29, the *Butte Miner* reported that a patrolman had discovered a man "wandering aimlessly on his hands and knees and apparently gravely ill" in the early hours of the morning. The man was taken to the emergency hospital, and it was determined he was not just intoxicated but "suffering from a serious attack of influenza aggravated by exposure."[159] Drunkenness and transience were not uncommon in Butte, but it's also possible that this unnamed man may have usually spent his nights in the warm backroom of a saloon, safe from the elements. There is no report of either his recovery or death.

Once both churches and saloons were closed, many families and individuals, especially linguistically and culturally isolated immigrants, had few options for community support. Their close neighbors often shared the same challenges but would offer what support they could with their own limited resources. While they may have helped limit the spread of influenza, orders to close churches and saloons also threatened to isolate a large number of Butte's residents and prevented them from obtaining much-needed assistance. The city's clergy and saloonkeepers understood this dilemma. While it's almost certain that many of the saloon and pool hall violations were due to businessmen trying to keep their incomes stable, it's just as likely that proprietors were doing what they and the clergy had always done—caring for the less fortunate members of their communities. Just as Reverend Brosnan and the religious community, saloon proprietors also suffered for their unwillingness to cease serving their communities. At least nine saloonkeepers and bartenders died of influenza in the last months of 1918.[160]

In many places around the nation, even in small, rural communities, people often abandoned one another during the pandemic—neighbors refused to check on each other, families starved because no one would bring them food in quarantine, and bodies piled up because undertakers were unwilling to handle any that potentially carried the influenza virus. While it's possible there were isolated incidents like this in Butte, the opposite is much more apparent. Officials ensured the families and individuals they placed in quarantine were not neglected. Business owners had to be forced to close shop, not due strictly to financial concerns but, as in the probable cases of many saloonkeepers, because they provided what many patrons couldn't get elsewhere—feelings of comfort and welcome. Residents clamored to attend funerals to pay their respects to friends and neighbors to the extent that they had to be ordered to stop so they wouldn't spread disease. Butte's undertakers formed an agreement to charge the same standard prices for the deceased, ensuring that human dignity in death came before price gouging and profiteering.[161] Many cities became ghost towns by choice, their residents afraid of catching the deadly infection. While the people of Butte were certainly very afraid, they still had to be forced into ghost town status. The old underground rule that Butte's miners had followed for decades also applied on the surface in the last weeks of 1918: Your life depends on the life of the man (or woman) next to you. If they live, so do you.

PART V

THE RECKONING

Our memories of this and other epidemics should not fail. Let us hope that through preparedness in health organization and in the education of new generations we may prevent a repetition of the terrific losses which influenza has cost.

—Dr. William F. Cogswell, "Tenth Biennial Report of the Montana State Board of Health for the Years 1919–1920"

Chapter 14

THE DEADLIEST HILL ON EARTH

Slowly, gradually, life in Butte returned to normal. The city's churches, theaters, and "places of amusement" were allowed to open.[162] Shops could advertise their sales in the newspapers again, and saloonkeepers brought their chairs back out. On December 14, Trevor Bowen of Washington Emergency Hospital decided, with the Butte–Silver Bow Board of Health's input, to accept no more patients. He estimated that the hospital could close by the end of the month. The worst was finally over.[163]

Time and distance allow the opportunity to see what public health officials may have had trouble recognizing in Butte in 1918. Now, given time to pore over records and with more knowledge and experience to decipher them, one can recognize that influenza in 1918 had preferences based on age, ethnicity, and gender. What didn't seem to matter to the disease, though, was occupation. Along with the clergy members and saloon proprietors, medical providers, teachers, clerks, hoteliers, students, soldiers, and housekeepers all succumbed to the disease. As the city's largest occupational group, it is no surprise that underground miners were responsible for the highest percentage of Butte's influenza deaths. In the best of times, the conditions underground were dangerous and challenging. The work was hard and deadly. Accidental injury and death were unfortunately common occurrences. Three of Butte's deadliest mining accidents occurred in the years before 1918, culminating with the 1917 Granite Mountain–Speculator Disaster. Miners often worked ten-to-twelve-hour shifts, hundreds to thousands of feet underground the entire time. Once a man went underground, only accident, illness, or injury was cause to bring him back to the surface before the end of shift.

Aside from the more obvious dangers of falling rock, misplaced explosives, fire, and pockets of poisonous gases, miners also contended with the unique health hazards working underground presented. Before the installation of ventilation systems in the 1920s, the air underground was stagnant, filled with the stench of perspiration, human waste, and animal excrement from the mules used to pull ore cars. Suffocating heat added to the conditions. Temperatures in the deepest underground areas easily reached 100 degrees Fahrenheit with a 100 percent humidity level. Steam rose from men's bodies as they came to the surface. Many would change clothing before returning home, but in Butte's freezing autumn and winter temperatures, sweat-soaked clothing could begin to ice over in the short walk from the mine shaft's entrance to the "dry room." All of these factors alone were cause for illness in Butte's underground miners, and in 1918, they also made it easier for influenza to take hold.[164] Miners could smell the stench in the air and feel its heat, but they were unaware of the number of other invisible dangers the mines' air carried. In a four-year investigation in 1908 through 1912, the Silver Bow County Board of Health found, among other infectious agents, *tuberculin* and *typhoid bacillus* in the air of the underground mines. The highest levels of these microbes were found in the driest levels of the mine, making it easier for them to spread. The dry areas had the most dust, and as the microbes dried, the dust carried them into the miners' airways. Additionally, silicate dust in the underground mines did irreparable damage to the lungs, increasing susceptibility to respiratory illness. A 1917–18 United States Public Health Service report estimated that "at least 20 per cent of the underground miners who had been employed five years or more in the Butte mines had miners' consumption."[165] Sensitive, already damaged respiratory and immune systems made many of Butte's miners more susceptible to influenza infection.[166]

Despite its unsanitary conditions and inherent dangers, working underground was, surprisingly, not the primary risk factor for influenza. Although underground miners were responsible for approximately 40 percent of the city's influenza mortalities, they made up about 37 percent of the population—a fairly well-balanced ratio. If spending half of their life underground made the miners more susceptible to the disease, a higher mortality rate compared to population should be expected. For a few months in the fall and winter of 1918, underground mining was no more dangerous than any other profession.[167]

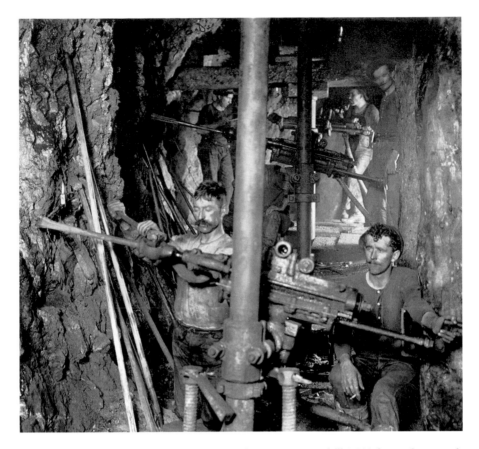

Notice the lack of safety equipment as these miners prepare to drill 1,900 feet underground. *Montana Historical Society.*

Butte itself—the smoky, rough, diverse, vibrant "Richest Hill on Earth"—was the single greatest risk factor its residents had of dying from influenza in 1918.

John and Annie Skubitz and their six children lived on Anaconda Road, in a Butte neighborhood now under the Berkeley Pit. Like nearly everyone else in Butte, the Skubitz family could probably see at least one of the city's giant headframes marking the entrance to a mine shaft from their front door. The Stewart, Parrot, Anaconda, and High Ore mines were nearby, and the Granite Mountain and Speculator sat right up the hill. The giant metal towers weren't the only visible reminder of Butte's primary industry. Before the Anaconda Smelter became operational in 1919, the smelting process was completed in Butte itself. Large fires burned day and night in and around the city, separating the valuable copper from the rocks pulled from the earth. A thick, constant haze hung over the city. The city's residents breathed in Butte's "sulphurous," acrid air each day whenever they stepped outside.[168] Annie would probably sometimes need to hold a rag over her face to filter the air when running errands, and it's quite possible that John occasionally had to carry a lantern in the middle of the day to help him see on the way to the saloon he operated. The Skubitz children played on dirt streets and in bare yards. They didn't climb trees because in Butte there were simply none to climb. Logging for timbers to frame underground tunnels had helped clear the surrounding mountains of trees, and the polluted smelter air had killed all vegetation in and around the city. There was no natural green anywhere in Butte. This environment was one of the main reasons that between 1911 and 1916, the city reported a mortality rate from tuberculosis more than double the national average. Hundreds of people in Butte, not just underground miners, suffered from lung diseases and infections. John Skubitz was one of them. He succumbed to pulmonary tuberculosis in the fall of 1913, shortly after Annie gave birth to their last child. Annie and the children stayed in the tiny house on Anaconda Road, surviving on a small Widows and Mothers pension Annie received and odd jobs she and the children could find.[169]

Along with polluted air, overcrowding and poor sanitation plagued all but Butte's most economically prosperous neighborhoods. Just blocks away from the wealthy neighborhood where Copper King William A. Clark had built his modern and extravagant mansion, small houses crowded onto the city's rocky slopes. It wasn't uncommon for entire families to live in one or two rooms. Due to overcrowding and the propensity to keep windows closed to keep polluted air out, ventilated indoor air space was incredibly limited. Many families may have kept a cow or some chickens in the yard. Milk or eggs would have been valuable to help feed the family and as extra income. Horses, cats, dogs, and the occasional cow or goat roamed the streets with no one bothering to clean up after them. Waste disposal was problematic, at best. In poorer neighborhoods, toilets were located outdoors and rarely tended. Refuse and stagnant water filled the dirt areas around homes. Though Annie Skubitz and her children had their own home, many young, single workers lived in crowded boardinghouses, often two or three to a single room. The boardinghouses had the same ventilation and waste disposal problems as single-family homes, often magnified due to the number of people living within them.[170]

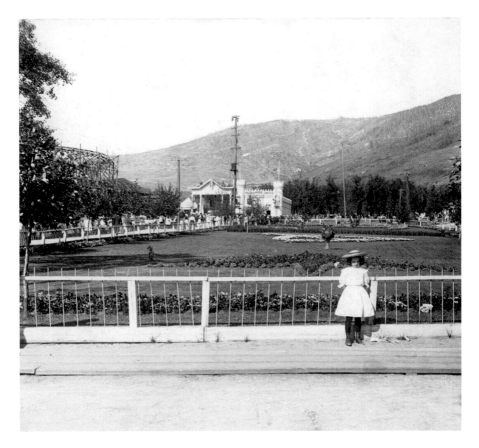

Pollution killed much of Butte's greenery and logging took the rest, as lumber was needed to frame underground mine shafts and tunnels. Heavily logged areas are visible on the mountains behind Columbia Gardens. *Montana Historical Society.*

In October 1918, just five years after John's death, tragedy befell the Skubitz house again. Annie contracted influenza, and for a couple of days, she probably struggled to keep up with her household chores. Finally, her older children would have realized their mother had no choice but to rest. Perhaps they helped put her to bed, pulling the blankets back over her when she kicked them off in a fit of fever and coaxing her into sitting up to sip water between coughing fits. When she developed pneumonia, the coughing would have changed. The dry hack would have grown thicker in the back of Annie's throat, and her breath, instead of rasping as it had, would have made gurgling and choking sounds.

There's no way to know how Annie would have felt when her seven-year-old son Leo began to complain of a headache. Did she worry that he would

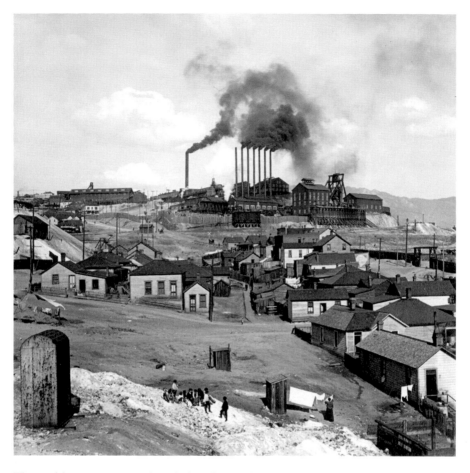

The smelting process poured smoke into Butte's skies at all hours of the day. *Montana Historical Society.*

become as sick as she? Did she try to comfort him, or was it impossible for her to hear his cries through her own pain and fevered delirium? His siblings would have laid him in the bed next to their mother—it may have been one of only two or three beds in the small house. Mother and son tossed with fever, shivering, sweating, and coughing. Little Leo also developed pneumonia. He may have been so sick that he didn't realize when his mother died in the bed next to him. He died the next day. The remaining five Skubitz children were alone and may have been among the number of Butte's children who became wards of the state that autumn and winter.[171]

The tragedies suffered by the O'Mearas, Muellers, Metzes, Reverend Brosnan, the Visnes, Vuciniches, Skubitzes, Sullivans, and so many other families and individuals in Butte made it clear, even early on, that no one was safe from influenza. Influenza's victims lived in various areas of the city: Centerville at the top of the hill; Dublin Gulch, just northeast of the business district; a row of boardinghouses in Finntown on east Broadway; primarily Italian Meaderville, now under the Berkeley Pit; the area around the railroad tracks where residents of all ethnicities found cheap rents; neighborhoods on the Flats in the area now around Interstate 90; affluent neighborhoods on the hill west of Montana Street where wealthy families lived in mansions with servants to attend their needs. But later, as it became apparent to epidemiologists that the virus preferred certain groups of people—young adults, men, recent immigrants—it also became clear that in Butte, influenza preferred some neighborhoods more than others. City officials may have begun to suspect as much. On November 15, the Red Cross suggested the Butte–Silver Bow Board of Health "investigate the Housing conditions of the rooming houses in the City and County" and "deputized" the city's doctors as "Sanitary officers" in order to give them more authority over the living conditions they encountered in their patients' homes.[172]

Though the board of health did not specifically mention any neighborhoods in its discussions of sanitation during the pandemic, an earlier study the board conducted on the city's sanitary conditions did. This 1908–12 study was undertaken in an effort to explain the city's high rate of tuberculosis. Officials inspected the mines and the sanitary conditions in many of the city's neighborhoods. Several of Butte's northeastern neighborhoods, including the Skubitzes', had especially high rates of tuberculosis and, officials discovered, often abysmal living conditions. As they compared their sanitation reports to records of tuberculosis deaths, the board made a discovery. Over 70 percent of all the deaths from tuberculosis recorded within Butte fell into an area roughly the shape of a Maltese cross. This area started just north of the railroad tracks, ran up the hill through Centerville, and encompassed much of the east end of Uptown Butte and beyond, including Finntown, Corktown, Dublin Gulch, and the Cabbage Patch. Areas in which the board had discovered the most crowded, dirty, and unhealthy living conditions were clearly within the cross's boundaries. Living conditions and tuberculosis were clearly linked.[173]

The other vital piece of information that can now be gleaned from this 1912 report is that living conditions not only affected tuberculosis mortality but influenza mortality rates as well. Approximately half of the city's influenza deaths in 1918 occurred within this area's borders in neighborhoods that housed not just underground miners but also bartenders, grocers, clerks, railroad men, and their families. The relationship between tuberculosis and influenza is significant and illuminating. Persons infected with tuberculosis were more likely to die of influenza than those who were not. Additionally, males were more likely to be infected with tuberculosis, and many of the neighborhoods within the boundaries defined in the 1912 report contained a large number of boardinghouses and hotels, which served as home for hundreds of Butte's young, single men. The highest rates were east of the Main Street dividing line, where most of the city's ethnic neighborhoods were located. Poor living conditions were influenza's strongest preference in 1918, and the concentration of young, male, and immigrant populations living within these unsanitary neighborhoods created the deadliest of all circumstances in Butte in the fall of 1918.[174]

INFLUENZA DEATHS WITHIN IDENTIFIED AREA

	Total	Immigrant	American-Born	Unknown
Total Mapped		230	250	30
Northeast	71	50	20	1
Southeast	79	42	30	7
Northwest	49	19	29	1

This study of Butte's susceptible neighborhoods also helps explain the discrepancy in mortality rates among immigrant groups. The board of health's report showed that living conditions and illness were undoubtedly linked. Butte's immigrants were more likely to live in the most crowded, unsanitary areas of the city, and this increased their risk for tuberculosis and other illnesses, including influenza. However, mortality rates among immigrant groups did not have even ratios when compared to population. For example, Butte's Finnish immigrants suffered a 4 percent mortality rate, while the city's larger Irish and English populations suffered mortality rates of 1 and 2 percent, respectively—a rate that matched that of the city's overall mortality rate of about 1.5 percent. In fact, though the Finnish were outnumbered by the Irish and English nearly three to one and two to one, 42 Finnish-born Butte residents died during the pandemic, compared to 45 Irish and 36 English immigrants. It's entirely possible that living conditions

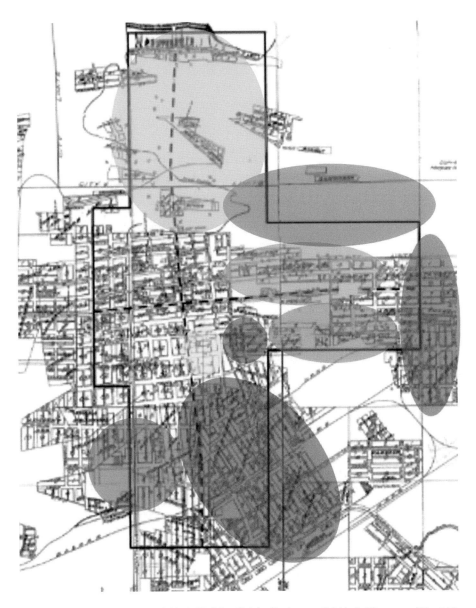

1: Centerville (Irish and Cornish); 2: Dublin Gulch, Corktown (Irish); 3: Finntown (Finnish);
4: Cabbage Patch (Irish); 5: Mixed Ethnic; 6: Red Light District; 7: Chinatown; 8: Serbian;
9: Mixed Ethnic. The Italian neighborhood of Meaderville is not pictured but lay east of
the neighborhoods labeled here in an area now under the Berkeley Pit and near the present-
day route of Interstate 15. *Author's collection.*

played a large role in this discrepancy. Many Finnish immigrants lived in incredibly crowded and unsanitary conditions. They "early formed their own community—three or four square blocks on East Granite and Broadway Streets, where boarding houses, saloons, stores, and…bathhouses soon predominated."[175] "Finntown" was contained within the area indicated by the board of health's sanitary report, and it is likely that at least some of its many boardinghouses were inspected and found lacking in proper sanitary measures. The Irish and the English, meanwhile, lived in various neighborhoods a bit more spread out within the city. Some of them fell in the indicated area, but others lay outside of it or were in areas of town that were less dense and crowded.

The city's Austrian population also seemed to suffer exponentially more than other groups during the pandemic, with a mortality rate of 7 percent. Unlike the Finnish, the Irish, or the English, though, there wasn't a specific neighborhood the Austrians claimed as their own. Like other immigrants from Central and Eastern Europe, the Austrians filtered through the city, settling in various areas and neighborhoods. If living conditions can't account for the Austrians' high mortality rate as it seemingly can for the Finnish, then what is to blame?

INFLUENZA DEATHS PERCENTAGE OF IMMIGRANT POPULATION

Data Set	Irish	English	Finnish	Austrian	German	All Other
Influenza Deaths	45	36	42	67	3	123
Total Population	3,196	2,181	1,013	955	858	4,677
Percentage	1%	2%	4%	7%	0%	3%

The culprit is probably impossible to prove, but immigrant mortality rates may also have been affected by specific place of origin. Many of Butte's Irish immigrants, for example, originally came from small cities and villages based on the mining industry. Upon arrival in America, they may have worked in mines in places like Pennsylvania, Michigan, and Colorado before making their way to Butte. The physical environment in most of these places was more similar to Butte's than those of the forests and farmlands in other parts of Europe. The Austrians, Finns, Italians, and Serbs were more

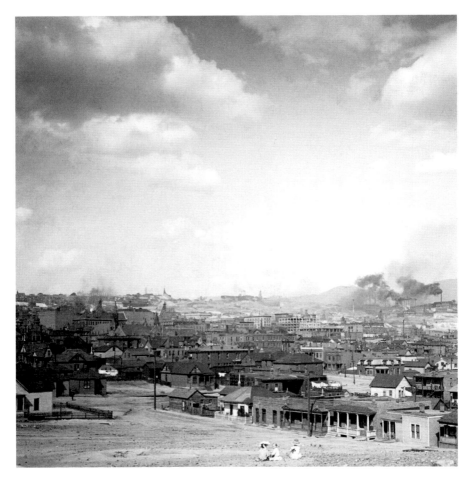

A view of one of Butte's crowded, working-class neighborhoods. *Montana Historical Society.*

likely to come from primarily rural, agricultural regions, whereas the Irish and English more often came from industrial areas where crowded living conditions and poor municipal sanitation were not uncommon. There, the chances of exposure to influenza and other pathogens were much higher than in isolated and rural communities. In short, the Irish and the English were often better adapted than their counterparts from Northern and Central Europe to living in a crowded and dirty city.

Yes, influenza had preferences, but it didn't discriminate. The O'Mearas lived just steps away from Clark's mansion in a wealthy, relatively clean neighborhood. The Metz family lived in one of the city's least crowded areas, and though Fred was born in Germany, Henry and Nellie Metz had both been born in Butte. Christian and Magdalene Visnes were from a small copper mining city. Yet influenza claimed them all. Regardless of where they were born and where they came from—the cities and tenement slums of the eastern United States, the mining camps of Colorado, the forests of Scandinavia, the rolling hills of central Italy, or the port cities of the British Isles—each of Butte's residents now had something in common: they lived in one of the most polluted cities in America. They walked down dirty, treeless streets and breathed acrid air in a city ringed by mountains they sometimes couldn't see through the smoky haze. When influenza struck, they all tried the same treatments and remedies, they prayed over the beds of the ill, and they wept at gravesides when their prayers went unanswered.

Chapter 15

THE PRIZEFIGHTER

B y January 1919, the Butte–Silver Bow Board of Health declared the influenza situation resolved. Though there were still some cases and infection was still a threat, board members decided to "notify the public through the 'press'…to use all precaution to guard against the disease."[176] Then it moved on to other discussion topics. The number of cases in the months immediately following was sporadic, and influenza took up no more of the board members' time than did other contagious diseases, like scarlet fever and diphtheria. The board of health estimated that approximately 5,700 people in the city had contracted the disease and about 640 had succumbed to it. Those numbers, though, are low. City records show over 700 deaths from influenza or influenza and pneumonia between October 1918 and January 1919. Countless residents probably never saw a doctor. Even when doctors were consulted, they were so overwhelmed with cases that it's likely many went unreported in their records and, consequently, to health officials. Some deaths, especially in the early days and weeks of the crisis, may have been attributed to something other than influenza. Deaths attributed to heart failure or lung congestion may have been due to preexisting conditions that influenza would have exacerbated but not taken the blame for.[177]

Approximately 130 people died of influenza in December, almost one-third fewer than the 304 deaths recorded in November, the pandemic's peak month. In the last week of 1918, 11 deaths were recorded, and as the new year began, the numbers began to taper off even further.

The influenza mortality rate was still higher than normal for January—the peak of the regular influenza season—and the mortality curve still reflected an abnormally high number of deaths in the twenty-to-forty-four age bracket. However, the total number of deaths wasn't enough for the board of health to continue justifying extreme control measures. The weekly, sometimes daily, meeting schedule board members had adopted during the crisis was replaced by the regular monthly agenda. By the end of February, the remaining cases of influenza "were mild in form and the majority of cases were among children," as is to be expected with seasonal influenza. The measures regarding funerals and the preparation of bodies were eased, and board members recommended that "all deaths occurring from Spanish influenza should be treated as other contagious diseases."[178]

The public health system is most effective when it learns from trying events, is willing to acknowledge its shortcomings, and uses the lessons learned to build a system for improvement. The same mistakes shouldn't be made twice. The changes the pandemic brought to the American public health system and public health in Montana were immediate, ongoing and effective. Prior to the pandemic, officials didn't require physicians to officially track or report cases of influenza. Now, though, they realized how deadly this regular, seasonal affliction could be and placed it on the same level as their other major concerns—diseases like diphtheria, tuberculosis, and syphilis.

Reporting incidences of a communicable disease allows public health officials to track the total number of cases, investigate how the disease may be spreading, and offer better guidance for mitigation. Had influenza been reportable prior to the pandemic, it's possible that public health officials would have identified it and put control measures in place much sooner. Controlling an outbreak is easier if it is identified before it has a chance to spread too far. After the crisis, state health officials required the reporting of influenza and, on Dr. Cogswell's recommendation, created a position for an "epidemiologist…for the purpose of studying the incidence of communicable diseases and co-operating with local and county health departments in the suppression of the same."[179] The epidemiologist position allowed for increased communicable disease reporting and more efficient and effective communication between local public health agencies around Montana and state officials in Helena. Subject matter experts could now provide more timely and accurate treatment and mitigation advice to protect the health of all Montanans.

EXCESS MORTALITY ᴵᴺ U·S·CITIES DURING INFLUENZA EPIDEMIC
PERCENT OF POPULATION DYING

CITY	SEPT. 8–NOV. 23 10 WEEKS	NOV. 24–FEB. 1 10 WEEKS	FEB. 2–MAR 29 8 WEEKS	TOTAL 28 WEEKS
PHILADELPHIA	.69	.01	.03	.73
FALL RIVER	.59	.05	.04	.68
PITTSBURGH	.59	.12	.06	.77
BALTIMORE	.57	.03	.0	.60
SYRACUSE	.55	.02	.02	.58
NASHVILLE	.55	.16	.12	.83
BOSTON	.50	.12	0	.62
NEW HAVEN	.49	.13	.0	.61
NEW ORLEANS	.49	.21	.0	.71
ALBANY	.48	.03	.02	.53
BUFFALO	.47	.10	.04	.61
WASHINGTON	.45	.12	.0	.54
LOWELL	.44	.10	.03	.56
SAN FRANCISCO	.42	.31	.02	.74
CAMBRIDGE	.39	.12	.0	.50
NEWARK	.38	.11	.04	.53
PROVIDENCE	.38	.13	.03	.53
RICHMOND	.35	.18	.02	.55
DAYTON	.33	.02	.03	.37
OAKLAND	.33	.22	.01	.56
CHICAGO	.32	.09	.04	.46
NEW YORK	.30	.09	.08	.47
CLEVELAND	.27	.11	.04	.42
LOS ANGELES	.27	.26	.01	.55
MEMPHIS	.25	.02	.09	.37
ROCHESTER	.25	.12	.03	.40
KANSAS CITY	.25	.27	.08	.60
DENVER	.24	.32	.07	.63
CINCINNATI	.22	.13	.11	.46
OMAHA	.22	.20	.0	.43
LOUISVILLE	.19	.04	.14	.37
ST. PAUL	.19	.13	.02	.34
COLUMBUS	.19	.15	.07	.41
PORTLAND	.18	.22	.03	.42
TOLEDO	.17	.02	.0	.17
MINNEAPOLIS	.17	.11	.07	.24
SEATTLE	.16	.16	.02	.36
INDIANAPOLIS	.15	.09	.08	.31
BIRMINGHAM	.15	.15	.0	.29
MILWAUKEE	.15	.18	.03	.37
ST. LOUIS	.12	.18	.04	.34
SPOKANE	.11	.13	.02	.25
ATLANTA	.07	.13	.0	.19
GRAND RAPIDS	.04	.12	.04	.19

Chart of excess mortality in U.S. cities during the influenza epidemic. Percentage of population dying of influenza in 1918–19, arranged by city. *National Museum of Health and Medicine.*

Through the spring of 1919, the number of disease reports increased over previous years, but deaths did not. Morbidity probably was not increasing; instead, reporting was now more accurate. The new disease surveillance and reporting measures seemed to be working. This system is still in place today. Healthcare providers are required to report all suspected or confirmed cases of communicable disease, including influenza, to local health departments. Local health officials follow up on all instances of disease, report these to the state health department, and work closely with healthcare professionals, with guidance from state epidemiologists, to recommend treatment, determine the cause of the disease, and mitigate the spread of infection.

The other, no less important change to the public health system in the months and years following the pandemic was its push to become more inclusive and to serve a more diverse population. Despite recent national movements for social activism and reform, public health and healthcare policies at the turn of the twentieth century were stuck in a Gilded Age mindset. A common belief was that the plights of the poor were of their own making, and the success of the country in general was more important than the individual. The upper classes believed that people living in slums and tenements were ill on a more frequent basis than their wealthier counterparts due not only to the conditions they lived in but also because of some flaw in their moral characters. The same personal faults that kept the poor in poverty also kept them from good health, or so the thinking went. "In the context of an epidemic," one researcher explains, "public health generally referred to a suite of measures designed to protect those elites from the contaminating influence of the disease-ridden rabble." Public health measures were aimed more at keeping social groups separated than preventing pathogenic invasions.

The pandemic of 1918 changed this perspective. Though it's true influenza was more prevalent in poorer neighborhoods, the rich and powerful were not completely spared. The O'Mearas, Muellers, and many more of Butte's wealthier families suffered as much as those in less-elite neighborhoods. According to the contemporary line of thinking, this was through no fault of their own. How, then, could it be the poor miner's fault that his family all took ill and many of them died? Public health officials saw firsthand that it was "no longer reasonable to blame an individual for catching an infectious disease" and that all cases of communicable disease needed the same care and treatment in order to protect not just a neighborhood but an entire city, state and nation.[180] Following the pandemic, countries around the world began to adopt government-funded public health and healthcare systems, allowing for better care of all the nation's residents, not just the wealthy. The groundwork was laid for the development of present public health and healthcare agencies like the World Health Organization, Centers for Disease Control and Prevention, and the United Kingdom's National Health Service.

In Butte, one of the Butte–Silver Bow Board of Health's main focuses in the years immediately following the pandemic was to improve the city's "sanitary conditions." The board increased the number of health inspectors, advocated for newer and improved sewage and waste disposal systems, and worked actively with members of the public to try to keep the city clean.[181]

Modern populations reap the benefit of these public health changes and advances today, but for countless families and individuals, life was forever changed after the events of 1918. With morbidity and mortality rates of approximately 15 and 2 percent, respectively, it's hard to imagine that there was anyone in Butte who didn't know someone who had been sick with influenza or died of the disease. Hundreds of families grieved the loss of a father, mother, brother, sister, or child. Rooms suddenly without occupants had to be cleaned out, and people all over the country and world received letters from Butte notifying them of the death of a friend or family member. The pandemic altered the natural course of life drastically for hundreds of families. Many lost the young men who were their primary breadwinners. Widows struggled to find work or left Butte altogether. Orphaned children were taken in by relatives in Butte, sent to live with family in other states, or became wards of the state. By November 1918, not even halfway through the crisis, the Butte–Silver Bow Board of Health had already taken over the care of fifty children whose parents were influenza victims. Many others required the same services by the time the pandemic was over.[182]

Influenza left indelible marks on entire communities, sometimes for years to come. Many of these were economic. Small businesses struggled to get back on their feet after days or weeks of lost revenue due to mandatory closures. In some instances, the shopkeepers, clerks, and maids who had opened the doors and helped keep businesses running died, leaving gaps in service. Conversely, while influenza may have financially devastated some families and businesses, a few communities around the nation experienced positive change in economic circumstances following the pandemic. Both influenza and World War I predominantly killed the demographic group that represented the manufacturing labor force—young, healthy men. Thus, cities with largely manufacturing-based economies experienced a rise in wages due to labor shortages. Wage increases were especially prevalent in cities with high influenza mortality rates. In Butte, young miners accounted for half of Butte's influenza deaths, and Montana's World War I combat mortality rate of 161 per 100,000 was the highest in the nation. Despite this, the mining industry in Butte did not experience the labor shortage and subsequent wage increases seen in other manufacturing-based cities like Pittsburgh and Cleveland.[183]

The mining industry was boom and bust, built on supply and demand. With the demand for copper at an all-time high due to the war in Europe, 1918 was an incredibly busy year for Butte's copper mines. During the "boom" portion of the cycle, more and more miners moved into town for work, creating a labor surplus. Additionally, industry issues like mine failures and labor disputes meant that there were always men looking for work in the mines. The transient nature of mining ensured that workers were always available to take the place of an ill, injured, or deceased miner, even when the deaths and illnesses were at record high numbers. John Gillie, manager of one of Butte's largest copper mines, the Anaconda, noted that workforce numbers didn't change throughout the course of the pandemic, even in the peak month of November, when hundreds fell ill and the number of deaths on some days reached double digits. The city's primary industry was responsible for many of its influenza deaths, but its transitory nature also ensured that the economic status quo remained unchanged during and after the social upheaval of the pandemic.[184]

Perhaps this is one reason why the pandemic largely remains forgotten, or at least ill-remembered, in Butte and other communities around Montana and the United States. At the Montana Nurses' Association Conference in July 1919, attendees paid tribute to nurses who had served overseas during the war, but influenza was not part of their discussion. Alice Becklin, an army nurse from Red Lodge, Montana, was stationed at Fort Riley, Kansas, during the pandemic—right near "ground zero," if the Haskell County, Kansas origin theories are true. Influenza, however, made little impression on Becklin. Years later, she remembered meningitis as a bigger issue. "The worst one [epidemic] I ever saw in my life was that meningitis….You got the flu and you died. You got meningitis and your head'd sit on your seat…. From meningitis we went to a measles epidemic and from measles they all got pneumonia and then pyemia [septicemia]."[185] Influenza, which took more lives than the other epidemics Becklin recalled combined, was only a passing comment.

You got the flu and you died.

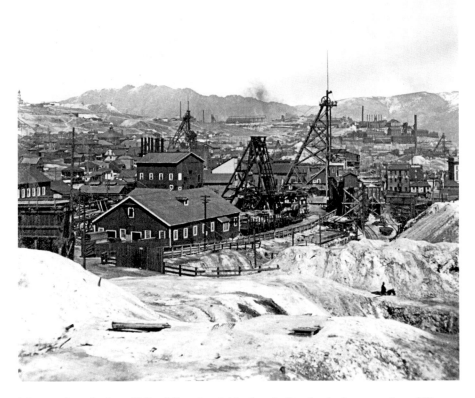

Mine yards sat in the middle of Butte's neighborhoods. Despite the large number of ill workers in 1918, mine workforce numbers remained unchanged. *Montana Historical Society.*

Perhaps because influenza killed so efficiently is why so few in the medical profession spoke of it in later years. In terms of successfully treating and mitigating the spread of the disease, doctors failed. This, of course, wasn't their fault; for many months, they simply had no idea what they were dealing with. Their previous knowledge and experience were useless in the face of this seemingly new and completely devastating pathogen. Rather than linger on these deficiencies, the medical profession chose instead to focus on its successes: advancements in battlefield medicine, such as blood transfusions and improved surgical practices, and the brave wartime service of thousands of doctors and nurses. Though they had been unable to control influenza, medical professionals took control of its narrative.

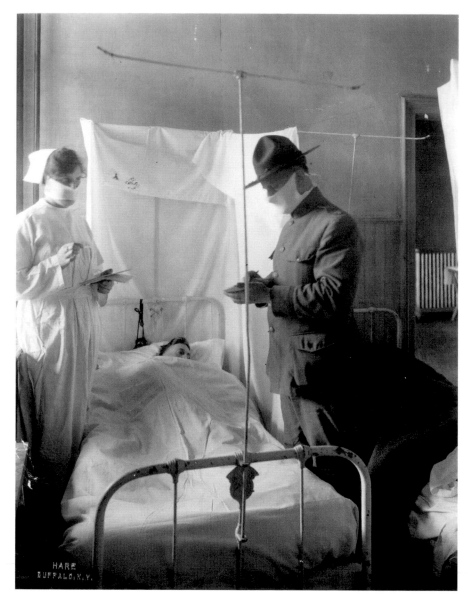

Army nurses cared for hundreds, if not thousands, of influenza patients, but many said little about their pandemic experience in the months and years immediately following. *National Archives.*

The general public followed suit. Influenza swept through their communities, uncontrollable and seemingly unstoppable, leaving devastation in its wake. Once it had gone, the people of Butte did not forget, but they chose to focus their remembrance around the positive, extraordinary, and, in their eyes, more controllable events of the age: their families and homes, victory overseas, the safe return of soldiers and the honorable sacrifices of those who did not come home, labor movements, women's suffrage, and Prohibition. In true Progressive fashion, Butte's residents relegated the pandemic to the past, allowing them to move forward with hope for the future. Like an Irish prizefighter throwing punches in front of a cheering crowd in a Butte saloon, the city took a hit, jumped up, wiped the blood away, and kept fighting.

Chapter 16
AFTER INFLUENZA

Time is measured not only in minutes, hours, days, and years but also in events. We delineate our lives based on what happens to us—before we finished school, after the birth of a first child, about the same time a loved one passed. It's hard to imagine that for those alive in 1918, influenza wouldn't be one of those markers, that life events weren't labeled BI or AI— Before Influenza or After Influenza.

Dr. William F. Cogswell had a long and distinguished career in public health and healthcare in Montana. In addition to his work improving communicable disease reporting and investigation, he continued studying tick-borne illnesses. Dr. Cogswell was a major player in the establishment of the Rocky Mountain Laboratory in Hamilton, Montana, today a National Institutes of Health biomedical research center specializing not only in the tick-borne illnesses that gave the lab its start but also in a number of emerging and re-emerging infectious diseases. His skill as a physician was well known, and he was respected throughout Montana. Dozens of fellow doctors attended his retirement ceremony, and the Blackfeet adopted him into their tribe, regarding him "not only as a great man but as a great healer."[186] He died in 1956 at the age of eighty-seven. "Many of Montana's existing public health rules and regulations, and public health programs had their initiation with Dr. Cogswell and many were sufficiently farsighted as to remain suitable for needs of today," Montana Board of Health secretary D.G.D. Carlyle stated in the wake of his predecessor's death. Today, the Montana Department of Public Health and Human

Service's Communicable Disease Epidemiology section is housed in the Cogswell Building.[187]

Dr. Jed Freund spent the rest of his life in Butte and died in 1932 at the age of fifty-seven after a long-term struggle with kidney and heart disease. He never married nor had children, instead devoting his life to the practice of medicine. He served as president of St. James Hospital Physicians on multiple occasions. His death was "received with extreme regret not only in hospital and medical circles but throughout the city and county."[188]

Dr. Walter C. Matthews continued practicing medicine in Butte and expanded his specialties to include laboratory and X-ray work after spending time at the Mayo Clinic in Rochester, Minnesota. His interest in radiography extended into photography, and he won local fame with a number of prints of the 1923 total solar eclipse. He died in Butte in 1924 at the age of fifty-five after a prolonged battle with cancer; the culminating event was complications following "an operation for the removal of a malignant growth." He left his wife, Pearl, and their daughters and mourners citywide, for "Dr. Matthews, always kind, generous, and cheerful…drew to him hosts of friends in this city [Butte] and elsewhere."[189]

Dr. Dan J. Donohue was a member of Butte's medical community and various civic organizations until his tragic death in 1929. After returning home from a late evening call, Dr. Donohue slipped and fell against his kitchen sink. Despite being attended by "a dozen medical men, the best Montana could provide," fifty-two-year-old Donohue never regained consciousness and died four days later. He was survived by his wife, Effie, and their three children.[190]

Dr. Caroline McGill served Butte for almost four more decades. In 1955, she received an honorary doctorate from Montana State College (now Montana State University) for "her outstanding service to Montana and the medical profession." She was only the second woman to receive the honor. Later that same year, the Butte Business and Professional Women's Club named her its "Woman of the Year" in recognition of her "achievements and unfailing assistance in worthy civic activities." A lifelong student and collector of Montana history, Dr. McGill, on two separate occasions, gifted historical collections to Montana State College. After leaving Butte, she settled in the Gallatin Valley and was laid to rest there after her death in 1957.[191]

Reverend Charles F. Chapman's name appeared in local papers hundreds of times after 1918. He presided over funerals, marriages, and many other services for Butte's residents as rector of St. John Episcopal

Church. In 1927, he was forced to resign his position due to ill health. He moved to Southern California in hopes that the milder climate would improve his condition. It did. The clergyman who "left Butte on a stretcher" took over as rector of St. Simon's Episcopal Church in San Fernando in 1930. He retired in 1932 and lived in Sherman Oaks, California, until his death in 1943. He was remembered in Butte as an "eloquent orator" and "outstanding figure" in civic activities.[192]

James Finlen had the Finlen Hotel torn down and rebuilt in 1923 for a cost of $750,000 (over $11 million today). The new Finlen quickly became one of Butte's finest establishments and hosted a number of notable persons over the years, including Charles Lindbergh, President Harry Truman, and then-senator John F. Kennedy. Later owners restored the grand hotel, and it still operates today in Uptown Butte in much of its former glory. Finlen himself served as vice president of Metals Bank and Trust and had a number of other business interests. He died in 1947 of a heart attack while on a pleasure trip in Nevada. Offering his hotel as an influenza hospital was apparently only one in a life of many charitable acts. Finlen was "the 'soul of charity,'" but he chose to keep many of his deeds quiet. "There are many persons in Butte today," the *Montana Standard* reported at his death, "who have been recipients of his generous charity but who did not know who their benefactor was."[193]

Dr. Huie Pock continued practicing his brand of Eastern medicine in Butte. When his wife died in 1923, in accordance with his traditional beliefs, Dr. Pock refused to have her buried in Butte. If she was not returned to her native village, the doctor believed, her soul would never find peace but roam the earth for eternity. Instead, the woman's body was placed in a glass-topped coffin and kept in the back of a funeral home. Dr. Pock visited her each day until his own death four years later. His body was placed into storage with his wife's, but sadly, disputes over his estate and the cost of shipping the bodies meant that Dr. and Mrs. Pock never made it back to China. For almost three decades, they lay in storage until the funeral home was sold. The bodies were turned over to the county, and their son paid for burial plots in Butte.[194]

Influenza traveled the globe again in the spring of 1919, though in a milder form than the months before, and it struck the *Mueller family* once more. Though Kathryn Mueller, Arthur's wife, had recovered from the illness in late 1918, it left her weak and in ill health. She traveled to New York City in hopes that "a lower altitude" would benefit her health. Rather, she again contracted influenza and in her weakened condition was unable to recover. She died in New York in June 1919. Arthur H. Mueller Jr. and his younger brother Charles lived with their grandparents when they were young. As a young man, Arthur studied medicine and volunteered to serve in the British American Ambulance Corps for the French forces in North Africa before the United States entered World War II. Tragically, Arthur never made it to his post. After almost a month with no word, his ship was declared lost at sea, and all passengers were pronounced deceased. Charles also served during and after the war years, working in embassies and consulates in South and Central America and East Asia. He returned to Montana, married, and had three children. He died in 1990 at the age of seventy-three.[195]

Young **Norman Visnes** was raised by his father's brother John. After graduating from Butte High School, Norman earned an engineering degree from the Montana School of Mines (now Montana Tech) and briefly served in the navy during World War II before going to work in mining, just as his uncle and father did. Norman moved through the ranks of the American Smelting and Refining Company, serving as general manager of the Northwest Mining Department in Wallace, Idaho; general manager of North American Mines in Tucson, Arizona; and, finally, American Smelting and Refining Company vice president at its headquarters in New York. The Montana School of Mines awarded him an honorary Engineer of Mines degree in 1966. Norman died in Coeur d'Alene, Idaho, in 1998 at age eighty-one and was survived by his wife, children, and grandchildren.[196]

Helen Jean Metz lived with her grandparents following the deaths of her parents. As a young woman, she moved out of her grandparents' home and worked as a seamstress in Butte before moving to Spokane, Washington, where she married in 1945. There is no record of her having children. Helen outlived her husband by over two decades and lived in Spokane until her own death in 1999. She was eighty-two.

After the deaths of their parents and infant brother, an uncle took the surviving **Vucinich children** to a remote Herzegovina village to live with extended family. The children, who had spent their entire lives to that point in America, grew up in a simple home without running water or electricity and tended livestock on the mountainsides. The eldest child, Wayne, moved to Los Angeles to live with his grandfather at age fifteen. He taught himself English and worked his way through school, eventually earning bachelor's, master's and doctoral degrees in Slavic languages and history from the University of California–Berkeley. After a brief stint with the U.S. government analyzing foreign affairs in the Balkans, Vucinich began a long and prestigious academic career at Stanford University. Affectionately known by students as "Uncle Wayne," Professor Vucinich taught courses on

Eastern Europe with passion and enthusiasm until 1988. He died in Menlo Park, California, in 2005.[197]

The *city of Butte* began to decline in population following the end of the First World War. Copper production, after its peak during the war, began to wane in Butte. Mining company consolidation resulted in the Anaconda Copper Mining Company dominating Butte—its mines and other institutions as interwoven as they all were with the copper business. Civil unrest stalked Butte for over two decades. Labor disputes continued through the 1930s, but the early 1920s were a particularly trying time. In 1920, a group of International Workers of the World protesters was shot by Anaconda Copper Mining Company guards, and the National Guard was called in to quell unrest—one of many times between 1914 and 1920. A labor strike in 1921 lasted ten months, and in 1923, a group of protesters attempted to use dynamite to blow up the Hibernian Hall.

The people of Butte were fighting for more than workers' rights during this time, though. Inspired by the strong nationalist sentiment, culminating with the Sedition Act of 1918, the Ku Klux Klan experienced growth and increased political influence throughout the United States in the years following the First World War. The group's reach was not restricted to the Southeast but stretched far into the nation, into the mountains, valleys, and plains of even the rural Midwest and Rocky Mountain regions. Many communities throughout Montana, possibly still feeling the war's social aftershocks, embraced the KKK's message of white Protestant supremacy. Butte, though, soundly rejected these ideas. Some unions refused to allow any members to claim KKK membership. Butte's large immigrant and Catholic populations were, naturally, opposed to any of the organization's messages and activities. Without much support, the KKK failed to establish a foothold in the state's largest city. Both the continued labor disputes and the stand against the KKK's message of hate are powerful illustrations of the proclivity of Butte's residents to stand up to powerful and intimidating forces in defense of their neighbors.

Dwindling copper output and increased industrialization made many mining jobs obsolete, and the city's population continued to decline. In the 1950s, the Anaconda Copper Mining Company moved from underground mining to the much less labor-intensive open pit mining and opened the infamous Berkeley Pit in 1955. The pit swallowed all of Meaderville and large parts of Dublin Gulch, Corktown, Finntown, and other neighborhoods on the east side of Butte. Houses, family-owned restaurants, saloons, and churches were demolished and the remains buried to make room for the expanding pit. The Berkeley grew each year, and by the 1970s, it began to encroach on the boundaries of Columbia Gardens. In 1973, the Anaconda Copper Mining Company announced the park's closure. Two months later, a fire ripped through the park's remaining structures, sparking rumors of company misdeeds. The whispers grew louder when the Continental Pit, another of the Anaconda Copper Mining Company's open pit mines, opened on the spot soon after. Mining continues today in the Continental, but the Berkeley Pit closed in 1982. Today, it's gradually filling with toxic wastewater and is part of one of the United States' largest Superfund sites.

Butte itself is, in some respects, unrecognizable from the bustling metropolis of one hundred years ago. The east end neighborhoods are now under open pit mines and toxic waste, and heavily traveled Interstates 90 and 15 merge and run through town with chain hotels and fast-food restaurants at their feet. The mine yards and headframes are still and quiet, and the smaller businesses in Uptown storefronts have changed hands and been renamed. Some of the more fortunate Victorian mansions on the West Side have been repainted and modernized. Others have sadly fallen into disrepair. Cars, trucks, and traffic signals have replaced the streetcar tracks. But Butte's residents refused to let change and modernization steal their city. They revitalized Uptown Butte, restoring many of its long-neglected, beautiful buildings and welcoming a new generation of business owners and residents. They embraced their city's history and worked to ensure it would never be forgotten. Uptown Butte is now one of the largest historic districts in the United States.

It's impossible that a disaster on the scale of the influenza pandemic of 1918 did not leave permanent marks on a community. Tragedy and sudden death bring family lineages to an abrupt halt and alter the course of life for orphaned children and widowed spouses. The orphan is made part of a new family with a different set of parents and siblings. The heartbroken widow or widower remarries and has more children. Loss gives life to a new generation. One hundred years after influenza, descendants of the men and women who fought the disease, who suffered from it, and who succumbed to it still call Butte home. Influenza is not only a part of Butte's history but also their legacy.

EPILOGUE

The enjoyment of the highest attainable standard of health is one of the
fundamental rights of every human being without distinction of race, religion,
political belief, economic, or social condition.
—Constitution of the World Health Organization

Brcvig Mission, Alaska, sits on the Seward Peninsula, overlooking the
Bering Strait's Port Clarence. In 1918, it was home to approximately
eighty people. The Inuit villagers received their supplies by dog sled
from the nearby village of Teller, which, in turn, was supplied by traders from
Nome, about sixty-five miles from Brevig Mission. This network is probably
how influenza got to Brevig Mission in 1918. Passed from person to person,
the virus moved from the cities of the western United States through the
Canadian Rockies, across the Yukon, and over the frozen tundra of central
Alaska. Between November 15 and 20, 1918, influenza killed seventy-two of
Brevig Mission's eighty residents—90 percent of the entire village.[198] Thirty-
three years later, microbiologist Johann Hultin visited Brevig Mission. His
purpose: acquire tissue samples from the bodies of influenza victims, buried
in the permafrost, frozen or partially frozen for the past three decades, in
hopes of bringing the virus within "back to life" to distinguish what made it
so deadly. His trip was ultimately unsuccessful; he was able to get the tissue
samples, but back in his Iowa lab, he was unable to revive the virus.[199]

In 1997, Hultin came across an article in *Science* magazine by Jeffery
Taubenberger, a molecular pathologist with the Armed Forces Institute of

Pathology. Taubenberger and his research partner, Ann Reid, had been attempting to revive the 1918 strain just as Hultin had years earlier, but their work was different in two ways: the samples and the science. Taubenberger and Reid were using samples stored in government facilities that had been obtained from military service members who had died of influenza—samples that didn't have the benefit of the natural "cold storage" of those Hultin found years before. Even with inferior samples, though, the equipment and knowledge Taubenberger and Reid had at their disposal, over forty years after Hultin, made it easier to identify fragments of the virus's DNA. However, they were unable to piece together the entire strand.[200]

Hultin thought he could help. On a mission funded with his own savings, the seventy-three-year-old microbiologist went back to Alaska and once again dug through the permafrost to open the mass grave he'd excavated over forty years earlier. Inside, Hultin found a specimen he thought was most promising: the preserved lungs of an obese woman, kept from decay by partially and completely frozen layers of fat. Hultin nicknamed the woman "Lucy" and sent Taubenberger her lungs. With Lucy's lung tissue, Taubenberger and Reid were able to reconstruct the entire genetic sequence of the deadly 1918 virus (an H1N1 strain).

This discovery wasn't only scientifically interesting but also incredibly important. Unlocking the virus's secrets increased the likelihood of discovering new ways to prevent and mitigate other potentially lethal strains of influenza. In the years since Taubenberger and Reid's discovery, researchers have identified that, excepting avian influenza viruses like H5N1, almost all influenza A cases are related to the 1918 virus—"descendants" of the deadliest influenza strain in recorded history.[201]

Shortly after Hultin's dig in Alaska, another team went searching for the remnants of the 1918 influenza virus in the permafrost of northern Norway. Residents of the Svalbard Islands, halfway between the Norwegian mainland and the North Pole, realized early in the twentieth century that their dead didn't decompose in the earth like in most other places in the world. Instead, the corpses of friends and loved ones froze and were preserved. Inspired by Taubenberger and Reid's work, a team of researchers decided to undertake the same mission as Hultin—acquire tissues from influenza victims and use them to isolate the 1918 virus. The team, led by Canadian scientist Kirsty Duncan, later appointed the country's first minister of science, was ultimately not as successful as they'd hoped. The Svalbard permafrost, and the bodies within it, had thawed and refrozen a number of times in the intervening decades, rendering the tissue samples far from perfect research

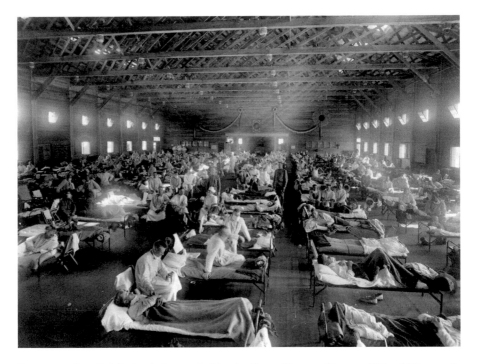

Emergency hospital during influenza epidemic, Camp Funston, Kansas. *National Museum of Health and Medicine.*

specimens. The bodies were soft and partially decomposed, their cellular structures damaged. Partial viral samples were extracted from the samples, but not enough to make a complete genetic sequence as Lucy's preserved organs had allowed Taubenberger and Reid.[202]

The searches for the 1918 influenza strain, on complete opposite sides of the globe, are perfect illustrations of how efficiently disease can spread. Even in 1918, when intercontinental travel took weeks instead of hours, deadly infection made its way around the globe, even to the most rural and isolated of communities. This point is more important today than ever before. More timely and accurate reporting methods, many developed in the pandemic's aftermath, help ensure that disease outbreaks do not go unnoticed until too late. Individuals diagnosed with a communicable disease can be treated quickly, their contacts identified efficiently, and control measures immediately put in place before the illness has a chance to spread any further. But in spite of public health's best surveillance and prevention efforts, disease outbreaks, epidemics, and pandemics are inevitable. As the population explodes, our world seems to shrink as crossing mountains, deserts, tundra, and vast oceans becomes quicker and easier, even necessary, as people constantly search for more space to call their own. These factors—growing population, ease of travel, climate change, and human encroachment into traditionally "wild" ecosystems—make the emergence, reemergence, and spread of communicable diseases unfortunately easy.

In 2016, anthrax spread throughout a region of northern Siberia. The outbreak began with a warm spell. The permafrost thawed and, with it, the carcass of a reindeer the disease killed decades before. The thaw allowed the bacteria, still alive, to reemerge and infect herds and people. Dozens of people were hospitalized and one child died. To mitigate the spread of disease, some families were evacuated and over two thousand reindeer were euthanized. But anthrax isn't the only disease that climate change can resurrect. Besides influenza and anthrax, scientists suggest there may be a whole host of "zombie" diseases hibernating in the permafrost—smallpox, bubonic plague, or viruses and bacteria that we have no knowledge of simply because they've been frozen for decades or even centuries. These pathogens may be different versions of the ones we're familiar with—a novel strain of influenza—or may be resistant to contemporary treatment methods. Perhaps they don't affect humans but instead prey on plant or animal life. They may not infect and kill large numbers of people but wreak havoc by disrupting ecosystems. Until the ground thaws—an inevitability with continued climate change—there's really no way of knowing exactly what is out there and how it might be fought.[203]

Ebola first emerged from the jungles of Central Africa in the late 1970s as humans forayed deeper into the continent's lush forests. Despite its wide spread in West Africa during the 2014 epidemic, fewer than ten cases appeared in the rest of the world, most in international healthcare aid workers. Vigilant monitoring systems put in place at international ports ensured that any traveler potentially exposed to Ebola was immediately placed under monitoring by a local public health department. In this way, public health systems, from the federal down to the local levels, were able to successfully control the spread of a deadly virus without disrupting entire communities. Stronger public health systems in West Africa may have helped identify and mitigate the epidemic much sooner and with substantially less loss of life.

Successful public health systems depend on strong infrastructure: clean water sources, municipal sanitation, and effective transportation and communication systems. When these fail or are nonexistent, old diseases that most of us in the First World relegate to decades and centuries in the past are given a chance to reemerge. In 2010, cholera took hold in the island nation of Haiti after a powerful earthquake devastated much of the island's infrastructure. Though it's now apparent United Nations aid workers brought the disease to the island, Haiti's damaged municipal and healthcare systems struggled to control and contain the outbreak. Cholera, the dread disease usually associated with nineteenth-century tenement slums, is now endemic in Haiti, sickens thousands of Haitians each year, and has killed more than eight thousand people. Natural disasters have the potential to cause outbreaks and epidemics wherever they occur—including developed nations—when the infrastructure and public safety systems that we typically take for granted are damaged or destroyed.

Fighting climate change, supporting local public health efforts, and lobbying for strong public safety systems are only the beginning. It is equally important to encourage the same measures around the world by maintaining a network of cooperative international public health systems and responses. In a world in which a deadly virus is only a few hours of flight time away from another country or continent, failing to contain a potentially deadly epidemic at its source allows it to spread around the world. Thus, part of a nation's duty in protecting itself from disease means using some of those resources to help protect others as well. The knowledge and experience the American public health system has gained over the last century, beginning with the important and painful lessons in 1918, are useless if we fail to share them. "We have to do multiple things to protect the health of the American people," says John Monahan, a former State Department special advisor for global health partnerships. "...One of them is investing in health security abroad."[204]

The world seemed smaller in 1918. So many of those who called Butte home waited days, weeks, and even months for information from families in other parts of the country and the world. Some spent their entire lives in the city as travel was too expensive, took too long, and was too unreliable. This dirty, smog-filled, beautiful, inimitable city, in the shadows of mountains, on a hill dotted with headframes, was their world. So when the pestilence struck in 1918, the people of Butte took in orphans, comforted widows, cared for the sick, and prayed for the souls of the dead. They used their resources to care for one another. Now, in our larger world, where we're connected on such a global level, where people, information, goods, and deadly pathogens can reach us in days, even hours, we must do the same. We can't pretend our world's health problems don't belong to us or someday, just as in 1918, they will.

NOTES

Prologue

1. "Disease Burden of Influenza," Centers for Disease Control and Prevention (hereafter CDC).
2. An *outbreak* is when more cases of a disease than normally expected are diagnosed in one defined area or season. An *epidemic* occurs when a disease is actively spreading within a geographic region. An epidemic becomes a *pandemic* when the disease has spread throughout an entire country or worldwide.
3. Kolata, *Flu*, 7.
4. Mullen and Nelson, "Montanans and the 'Most Peculiar Disease.'" It wasn't until late 1918, at the height of the pandemic, that the Montana State Board of Health began requiring physicians to report cases of the disease. Even then, the board suspected that, due to overwork or clerical oversight, physicians still didn't report all cases. Thus, Montana's mortality rate may have been higher than officially reported.
5. Ibid., 55. The number of victims is based on estimates from City of Butte and Silver Bow County vital records. Though the City of Butte recorded 707 deaths, Silver Bow County recorded more in the areas bordering city limits. This puts the total for the immediate region at about 1,000. In all likelihood, the actual number was probably higher, as many deaths went unreported or were misattributed to other causes. In "Montanans and the 'Most Peculiar Disease,'" Mullen and Nelson estimate that Butte was responsible for one-third of Montana's pandemic mortalities.

Chapter 1

6. Hoffman, "Mining History of Butte."
7. Kearney, *Butte Voices*, 91, 94, 97. Hennessey's, the Pekin Noodle Parlor, the M&M Bar and a number of other Uptown businesses are still in operation in some form today. The Hennessey Building houses the Hennessey Market on its first floor and luxury apartments on its upper floors. The Metals Bank Building is home to Metals Bar and Grill, the Park and Main Café, an art gallery, a salon and condominiums. Dozens of other Uptown retail spaces have been converted into new spaces.
8. United States Census Bureau, 1910 Census, Silver Bow County, MT; Murphy, *Mining Cultures*, 23.
9. Kearney, *Butte Voices*, 170.
10. Ibid., 194–95.
11. Ibid., 181.
12. Ibid., 185, 168.
13. Ibid., 211, 213–14.
14. Ibid., 171.
15. Ibid.
16. Ibid., 173–75. Several other neighborhoods not discussed here were also part of early twentieth-century Butte. Two that still exist today are Walkerville and the Flats. Together, these two areas serve as bookends for Butte, bordering the city on the north and south. Walkerville sits north of Centerville just outside the city limits. To get to Walkerville, one crested the summit of Butte's hill. This makes Walkerville often several degrees warmer than Butte proper in the winter, as the colder air is trapped in the valley below. Walkerville had its own shops and municipal services. The Flats begins at the southern end of Central Butte, stretching out along the valley floor for almost nine miles toward the mountains. In Butte's earliest days, the neighborhood was home to Native Americans. As the mining industry grew, so did the Flats, eventually becoming a primarily working-class neighborhood of mixed ethnicity. Walkerville and the Flats play minor roles in the story of the 1918 influenza pandemic in Butte compared to the areas described above.
17. "Thanks to Bravery of 2 Men, 31 Butte Miners Made It Out Alive," *Montana Standard*, June 8, 2017. For a detailed and gripping account of the Granite Mountain–Speculator Disaster of 1917, see Punke, *Fire and Brimstone.*

Chapter 2

18. Barry, *Great Influenza*, 93–94.
19. Crosby, *America's Forgotten Pandemic*, 19.
20. Ibid., 25–27, 28.
21. Ibid., 28, 25–26.

Chapter 3

22. Influenza C viruses do infect humans but usually only cause mild respiratory illnesses. For the most part, scientists believe they do not cause epidemics. Influenza D viruses are not known to infect people but are primarily found in cattle.
23. The influenza virus responsible for the 1918 pandemic was also an H1N1 strain, and H1N1 causes infections now nearly every flu season. In the decades since 1918, humans have developed some level of natural immunity to H1N1.
24. "Types of Influenza Viruses," CDC.
25. "Influenza A Type Viruses," CDC; "Avian Influenza A Virus Infections in Humans," CDC; "Highly Pathogenic Asian Avian Influenza A (H5N1) Virus," CDC.
26. "Key Facts about Human Infections with Variant Viruses," CDC.
27. "How the Flu Virus Can Change: 'Drift' and 'Shift,'" CDC.

Chapter 4

28. Death Certificate for Michael Murtha, October 4, 1918, File No. 24502, City of Butte, Butte–Silver Bow Public Archives (hereafter BSBPA), Butte, MT.
29. Butte City Directories, 1914, 1916, 1917, BSBPA, Butte, MT.

Chapter 5

30. "Viola Paus Passes Away After a Week's Illness," *Scobey Sentinel*, September 27, 1918.
31. *River Press*, October 16, 1918.

32. Montana State Board of Health Records, Record Series 238, Box 1, Folder 2, October 9, 1918, Montana Historical Society Research Center (hereafter MHSRC), Helena; *Great Falls Tribune*, May 27, 1956.

33. *River Press*, October 16, 1918.

34. Montana State Board of Health Minutes, October 9, 1918, Montana State Board of Health Records, Record Series 238, Box 1, Folder 2, MHSRC, Helena.

35. Butte City Directories, 1917, BSBPA, Butte, MT; *Montana Standard*, February 4, 1932.

36. *Independent Record*, October 4, 1929; *Montana Standard*, October 4, 1929.

37. Montana State Board of Health Minutes, October 9, 1918, Montana State Board of Health Records, Record Series 238, Box 1, Folder 2, MHSRC, Helena.

38. *Butte Miner*, October 17, 1924; Butte City Directories, 1918, BSBPA, Butte, MT.

39. Butte Health Officer, Department of Health Minute Book, 1903–1923, October 9, 1918, Silver Bow County Board of Health Collection, GR.HL. SB.002, Box 1, Volume 1, BSBPA, Butte, MT.

40. *Montana Standard*, March 23, 1943.

41. Butte Health Officer, Department of Health Minute Book, 1903–1923, October 11, 1918, Silver Bow County Board of Health Collection, GR.HL.SB.002, Box 1, Volume 1, BSBPA, Butte, MT.

42. Ibid.

43. Ibid.

44. Ibid.

45. Ibid.

46. Ibid., October 21, 1918.

47. Ibid., October 30, 1918.

48. Ibid., October 18, 19, 31, 1918.

49. "Police Guard at Funerals," *Anaconda Standard*, October 23, 1918.

50. Butte Health Officer, Department of Health Minute Book, 1903–1923, October 12, 15, 22, 1918, Silver Bow County Board of Health Collection, GR.HL.SB.002, Box 1, Volume 1, BSBPA, Butte, MT.

51. Ibid., October 22, 1918.

52. Ibid., October 11, 1918.

53. Ibid., October 21, 1918.

54. Ibid.

55. This is one instance in which the numbers provided by health authorities do not match the death records. It's possible that some of the deaths the

doctors referred to were recorded by Silver Bow County instead of the City of Butte. As the pandemic response continued into the late fall and winter, health authorities would discuss the need to combine vital records of the city and county to keep better track of numbers like these.

56. Butte Health Officer, Department of Health Minute Book, 1903–1923, October 15, 18, 1918, Silver Bow County Board of Health Collection, GR.HL.SB.002, Box 1, Volume 1, BSBPA, Butte, MT; Death certificate for Mrs. Charles McDonald, October 16, 1918, File No. 24132, City of Butte, BSBPA, Butte, MT.

57. Butte Health Officer, Department of Health Minute Book, 1903–1923, October 21, 1918, Silver Bow County Board of Health Collection, GR.HL.SB.002, Box 1, Volume 1, BSBPA, Butte, MT

58. Death Certificates, City of Butte, BSBPA, Butte, MT.

Chapter 6

59. Mullen and Nelson, "Montanans and the 'Most Peculiar Disease.'"

60. Today, public health departments are staffed by nurses, epidemiologists and other subject matter experts. The local board of health consists of various community leaders, which may include government officials, school representatives and healthcare providers. In the state of Montana, each local board of health must designate a medical officer—a physician who oversees all medical aspects of the public health department's activities. The medical officer, for instance, will sign standing orders allowing the health department's nurses to provide immunizations and certain medical treatments without a physician physically on-site.

61. Eyler, "State of Science."

62. Mullen and Nelson, "Montanans and the 'Most Peculiar Disease,'" 59.

63. Barry, *Great Influenza*, 242.

64. "Great Epidemic Caused by Present War Diet," *Anaconda Standard*, October 18, 1918.

65. Crosby, *America's Forgotten Pandemic*, 216; Quinn, *Flu: A Social History*, 139.

66. Eyler, "State of Science."

67. "Types of *Haemophilus influenza* Infections," CDC.

68. "The Medical and Scientific Conceptions of Influenza."

69. "Uncle Sam's Advice on Flu," *River Press*, October 23, 1918.

70. Ibid.

71. Ibid.

72. Ibid.

73. Ibid.

74. Ibid.

75. "Propaganda for Reform," 1763.

76. Eyler, "State of Science."

77. Butte Health Officer, Department of Health Minute Book, 1903–1923, October 18, 1918, Silver Bow County Board of Health Collection, GR.HL.SB.002, Box 1, Volume 1, BSBPA, Butte, MT.

78. Ibid., October 18, 1918; November 3, 1918.

79. Ibid., November 4, 1918

80. Ibid.

81. *River Press*, October 23, 1918.

82. Ibid., October 16, 1918; Eyler, "State of Science."

83. "Gave Her Own Life that Others Might Live," *Butte Miner*, November 2, 1918.

84. American Red Cross Butte Chapter, "How to Avoid Influenza and Other Sickness," *Anaconda Standard*, October 23, 1918.

85. Butte Health Officer, Department of Health Minute Book, 1903–1923, October 20, November 9, 1918, Silver Bow County Board of Health Collection, GR.HL.SB.002, Box 1, Volume 1, BSBPA, Butte, MT.

86. Ibid., October 23, 1918.

87. *Butte Miner*, October 24, 1918.

88. *Anaconda Standard*, October 23, 1918; *Butte Miner*, October 24, 1918.

89. *Butte Miner*, October 24, 1918.

90. Butte Health Officer, Department of Health Minute Book, 1903–1923, October 23, 24, 1918, Silver Bow County Board of Health Collection, GR.HL.SB.002, Box 1, Volume 1, BSBPA, Butte, MT.

91. "Transform School House into 'Flu' Hospital," *Butte Miner*, October 25, 1918.

92. Ibid., October 24, 26, 28, 1918.

93. Ibid., October 28, 1918.

94. Ibid., November 29, 1918.

95. "Spanish 'Flu' Is Not a Joke," *Butte Miner*, October 19, 1918.

Chapter 7

96. *Anaconda Standard*, October 24, 1918.

97. Ibid.

98. *Butte Miner*, October 25, 1918.

99. Death Certificates for Patrick Sullivan, October 26, 1918, File No. 24343; Peter Sullivan, October 27, 1918, File No. 24398; Michael Sullivan, November 2, 1918, File No 24396; "Patrick Casey Succumbs," *Anaconda Standard*, October 28, 1918.

100. Death Certificates for Emma Duffy, October 18, 1918, File No. 24146; Frank Duffy, October 23, 1918, File No. 24233; Daniel Sheedy, October 24, 1918, File No. 24426; Daniel Sheedy, October 24, 1918, File No. 24425; Frances McLaughlin, October 20, 1918, File No. 24175; Rose McLaughlin, October 22, 1918, File No. 24195, City of Butte, BSBPA, Butte, MT.

Chapter 8

101. Punke, *Fire and Brimstone*, 5.

102. Ibid.

103. Butte Health Officer, Department of Health Minute Book, 1903–1923, October 28, 1918, Silver Bow County Board of Health Collection, GR.HL.SB.002, Box 1, Volume 1, BSBPA, Butte, MT.

104. Ibid., October 26, November 3, 4, 1918; "Another Saloon Violation," *Anaconda Standard*, November 5, 1918.

105. Butte Health Officer, Department of Health Minute Book, 1903–1923, November 8, 1918, Silver Bow County Board of Health Collection, GR.HL.SB.002, Box 1, Volume 1, BSBPA, Butte, MT.

106. Ibid., November 8, 14, 1918.

107. Coburn, Wagner and Blower, "Modeling Influenza Epidemics."

108. Butte Health Officer, Department of Health Minute Book, 1903–1923, November 15, 1918, Silver Bow County Board of Health Collection, GR.HL.SB.002, Box 1, Volume 1, BSBPA, Butte, MT.

Chapter 9

109. Ibid., November 14, 1918.

110. Montana Code Annotated 50-2-116, 2017.

111. Ibid.

112. Administrative Rules of Montana 37.114.307, 2017.

113. Butte Health Officer, Department of Health Minute Book, 1903–1923, November 22, 1918, Silver Bow County Board of Health Collection, GR.HL.SB.002, Box 1, Volume 1, BSBPA, Butte, MT.

114. Ibid., November 28, 1918.

115. Ibid.

116. "Doctors Urge a Quarantine," *Butte Miner*, November 18, 1918.

117. "Dr. Caroline McGill: Mining City Doctor," VF0592, BSBPA, Butte, MT.

118. "Doctors Urge a Quarantine," *Butte Miner*, November 18, 1918.

119. Ibid.

120. Butte Health Officer, Department of Health Minute Book, 1903–1923, November 20, 22, 1918, Silver Bow County Board of Health Collection, GR.HL.SB.002, Box 1, Volume 1, BSBPA, Butte, MT.

121. Ibid., November 25, 1918.

122. Ibid., November 19, 1918.

123. Ibid., November 29, 1918.

124. Ibid., November 30, 1918.

125. *Butte Miner*, November 16, 1918.

126. Butte Health Officer, Department of Health Minute Book, 1903-1923, December 4, 1918, Silver Bow County Board of Health Collection, GR.HL.SB.002, Box 1, Volume 1, BSBPA, Butte, MT.

127. Ibid., November 30, 1918.

128. Now it's understood that contracting influenza from the dead body of one of the disease's victims is highly unlikely, as influenza is spread primarily through respiratory means. To be infected from a dead body, one would have to touch the mucous of the dead person, then touch his or her own eyes, nose, or mouth. The virus will only survive in a dead host, or in an environment without a living host, for about twenty-four hours, at most.

129. Butte Health Officer, Department of Health Minute Book, 1903–1923, November 21, 1918, Silver Bow County Board of Health Collection, GR.HL.SB.002, Box 1, Volume 1, BSBPA, Butte, MT.

Chapter 10

130. Vigsnes Mine Museum; Petition for Naturalization for Christian Visnes, May 9, 1905, Petition No. 984; Death Certificates for Chris Visnes, November 7, 1918, File No. 24547; Madeline Visnes, November 11, 1918, File No. 24562, City of Butte, BSBPA, Butte, MT.

131. Death Certificates for Chris Visnes, November 7, 1918, File No. 24547; Madeline Visnes, November 11, 1918, File No. 24562, City of Butte,

BSBPA, Butte, MT; Burial Record for Chris Visnes, November 10, 1918, ID File No. 4238, Mt. Moriah Cemetery, Butte, MT, BSBPA, Butte, MT; United States Census Bureau, 1930 Census, Butte, Montana.

132. Katz, "Influenza 1918: A Study in Mortality," 416; Luk, Gross and Thompson, "Observations on Mortality," 1376.

133. Any mortality rates for age, gender and ethnic groups were calculated using two sources: the City of Butte's death certificates for September 1918 through February 1919 (the months of the pandemic's height in Butte) and the 1910 census. During this time, 707 deaths were recorded that list influenza as either the primary cause or a contributing factor of death. These 707 deaths are not a total of Butte's pandemic deaths (others were filed with Silver Bow County), but they provide a sample statistically large enough for comparison to the whole with a confidence factor of 95 percent and a margin of error of less than 5 percent. When looking at individual factors like age and gender, the numbers may not add up to 707, as not all records listed these specific demographic factors. However, each individually cited trait is listed enough times to keep figures statistically significant at the rates listed above. Records from the 1910 census were used to calculate ratios of influenza deaths to total population. Though taken eight years prior to the pandemic, the census is the most complete and accurate contemporary population information available and the best means of calculating mortality rates within the city. This mortality curve and all other graphics and illustrations regarding mortality rates were created by the author. Materials utilized in their creation are cited where necessary. United States Census Bureau, 1910 Census, Montana.

134. Barry, *Great Influenza*, 249–51; Quinn, *Flu*, 156; Byerly, *Fever of War*, 126.

135. Garret, "War and Pestilence," 713; Phillips and Killingray, introduction to *The Spanish Influenza Pandemic*, 8; Davies, *Devil's Flu*, 37; United States Census Bureau, 1910 Census, Montana.

Chapter 11

136. Death certificates, City of Butte, BSBPA, Butte, MT.

137. Barry, *Great Influenza*, 408; C.E. Winslow and J.F. Rogers, "Statistics of the 1918 Epidemic of Influenza in Connecticut," *Journal of Infectious Disease* 26 (1920): 185–216, as cited in Katz, "Influenza 1918: A Further Study in Mortality," 619.

138. Walters, "Influenza 1918," 857; Katz, "A Study in Mortality," 422; Katz, "Influenza 1918: A Further Study in Mortality," 619; United States Census Bureau, 1910 Census, Montana.

139. "The Story of the Bohunk," *Butte Evening News*, July 24, 1910, from Writers' Project of Montana, *Copper Camp*, 140–41.

140. Spiro Vucinich listed Austria as his birthplace on his 1902 naturalization papers. However, his death certificate lists his birthplace as Herzegovina. Herzegovina was still part of the Austro-Hungarian Empire when Spiro was naturalized. The empire broke up in 1917, and Herzegovina's official status was in limbo at the time of Spiro's death. In December 1918, Herzegovina became part of the Kingdom of Yugoslavia.

141. *Butte Miner*, November 27, 1918. Death certificates for Veleko Vucinich, November 21, 1918, File No. 25002; Spiro Vucinich, November 26, 1918, File No. 24943; Soka Vucinich, November 27, 1918, File No. 24942; Naturalization Records, K-N, 1890–1904, MHSRC, Helena; U.S. City Directories, 1918, Los Angeles; "Wayne S. Vucinich, Father of East European Studies, Dead at 91," Stanford News Service.

142. Death certificates for Clementina Marianetti, October 22, 1918, File No. 24691; Pablo Zarragoitia, October 19, 1918, File No. 24493; Gertrude Sithes, October 20, 1918, File No. 24152; Emil Sjoguist, December 17, 1918, File No. 25135; Edward O'Rourke, November 24, 1918, File No. 24726, City of Butte, BSBPA, Butte, MT.

Chapter 12

143. Steele, "Flu Epidemic of 1918," 85–86.

144. Waldrup, "Huie Pock," 4.

145. Ibid.

146. Ibid.

147. "Names and Faces," Mai Wah Society.

148. Everett, "Butte's Far Eastern Influences."

Chapter 13

149. Butte Health Officer, Department of Health Minute Book, 1903–1923, December 5, 1918, Silver Bow County Board of Health Collection, GR.HL.SB.002, Box 1, Volume 1, BSBPA, Butte, MT.

150. Ibid., December 7, 1918.

151. "Ministers Protest," *Anaconda Standard*, October 11, 1918.

152. Emmons, *Butte Irish*, 97.

153. Brosnan, personal letter, February 18, 1917, VF0234, BSBPA, Butte, MT.

154. *Butte Miner*, November 11, 1918.

155. *Montana Standard*, July 21, 1996.

156. Writers' Project of Montana, *Copper Camp*, 1.

157. "Saloonman Held for Selling Over a Bar," *Anaconda Standard*, October 26, 1918.

158. Emmons, *Butte Irish*, 42–43; Writers' Project of Montana, *Copper Camp*, 87–88.

159. *Butte Miner*, November 29, 1918.

160. Emmons, *Butte Irish*, 42–43; Writers' Project of Montana, *Copper Camp*, 87–88; "Saloonman Held for Selling Over a Bar," *Anaconda Standard*, October 26, 1918; Butte Health Officer, Department of Health Minute Book, 1903–1923, November 4, 5, 1918, Silver Bow County Board of Health Collection, GR.HL.SB.002, Box 1, Volume 1, BSBPA, Butte, MT; Death certificates, City of Butte, BSBPA, Butte, MT.

161. "Board Receives but One Bid for Burying Paupers," *Anaconda Standard*, December 22, 1918.

Chapter 14

162. Butte Health Officer, Department of Health Minute Book, 1903–1923, November 8, 1918, Silver Bow County Board of Health Collection, GR.HL.SB.002, Box 1, Volume 1, BSBPA, Butte, MT.

163. Ibid., December 18, 1918.

164. Silver Bow County, "Report of Investigation," 11, 14; Murphy, *Mining Cultures*, 12, 16.

165. Toole, *Twentieth-Century Montana*, 147.

166. Silver Bow County, "Report of Investigation," 15.

167. Death certificates, City of Butte, BSBPA, Butte, MT.

168. Howard, *Montana*, 97.

169. Death certificates, City of Butte, BSBPA, Butte, MT; Widows and Mothers Pensions, BSBPA, Butte, MT; Emmons, *Butte Irish*, 72; Murphy, *Mining Cultures*, 4.

170. Silver Bow County, "Report of Investigation"; Emmons, *Butte Irish*, 73.

171. Death certificates, City of Butte, BSBPA, Butte, MT.
172. Butte Health Officer, Department of Health Minute Book, 1903–1923, November 15, 30, 1918, Silver Bow County Board of Health Collection, GR.HL.SB.002, Box 1, Volume 1, BSBPA, Butte, MT.
173. Silver Bow County, "Report of Investigation," 18–19; Silver Bow County, "Report Showing Result of Inspection of Dwellings, Hotels? (sp) Rooming Houses and Boarding Houses and Their Surroundings," in Silver Bow County, "Report of Investigation."
174. Noymer and Garenne, "1918 Influenza Epidemic's Effects," 565.
175 Writers' Project of Montana, *Copper Camp*, 128.

Chapter 15

176. Butte Health Officer, Department of Health Minute Book, 1903–1923, January 8, 1919, Silver Bow County Board of Health Collection, GR.HL.SB.002, Box 1, Volume 1, BSBPA, Butte, MT.
177. Ibid., January 8, 1919.
178. Ibid., February 22, 1919.
179. Cogswell, "Ninth Biennial Report," 1.
180. Spinney, "How the 1918 Flu Pandemic Revolutionized Public Health."
181 Butte Health Officer, Department of Health Minute Book, 1903–1923, Silver Bow County Board of Health Collection, GR.HL.SB.002, Box 1, Volume 1, BSBPA, Butte, MT.
182. "Health Board Provides Care for Children Left Destitute by Epidemic," *Anaconda Standard*, November 2, 1918.
183. Howard, *Montana*, 203.
184. Garrett, "War and Pestilence"; "Methods to Combat the Raging Epidemic Are Being Defined," *Anaconda Standard*, October 22, 1918; Emmons, *Butte Irish*, 135.
185. Becklin, interview with Wallis.

Chapter 16

186. *Great Falls Tribune*, May 27, 1956.
187. Ibid.
188. *Montana Standard*, February 4, 1932.
189. *Butte Miner*, October 17, 1924.

190. *Montana Standard*, October 4, 1929.
191. Ibid., February 5, 1957, 3.
192. Ibid., March 23, 1943; *Los Angeles Times*, February 8, 1930.
193. *Montana Standard*, March 20, 1947.
194. Waldrup, "Huie Pock," 5–6.
195. *Anaconda Standard*, June 21, 1919; *Montana Standard*, May 20, 1941; *Montana Standard*, December 29, 1990.
196. *Montana Standard*, May 15, 1966, August 25, 1998.
197. Taylor, "Wayne Vucinich."

Epilogue

198. Rozell, "Villager's Remains."
199. Ibid.
200. Ibid.
201. Ibid.; "Jeffery Taubenberger," Killer Flu, Public Broadcasting Service, www.pbs.org/wnet/secrets/jeffery-taubenberger/223/; Taubenberger and Morens, "1918 Influenza."
202. McKenna, "Canada's First (and Female) Science Minister Is a Badass."
203. Doucleff, "Anthrax Outbreak in Russia"; Meyer, "Zombie Diseases of Climate Change."
204. Yong, "Deadly Panic-Neglect Cycle."

BIBLIOGRAPHY

Primary Sources

Administrative Rules of Montana. 37.114.307. 2017.

Anaconda Standard (Butte, MT).

Becklin, Alice. Interview by Trudy Wallis. Personal interview. Red Lodge, MT, October 5, 1975. Montana Historical Society Research Center, Helena, MT.

Brosnan, Rev. Patrick. Personal letter. February 18, 1917. VF0234. Butte–Silver Bow Public Archives, Butte, MT.

Butte City Directories. Butte–Silver Bow Public Archives, Butte, MT.

Butte Health Officer. Department of Health Minute Book, 1903–1923. Silver Bow County Board of Health Collection. GR.HL. SB.002. Butte–Silver Bow Public Archives, Butte, MT.

Butte Miner (Butte, MT).

City of Butte. Death Certificates. Butte–Silver Bow Public Archives, Butte, MT.

Cogswell, W.F. "Ninth Biennial Report of the State Board of Health for 1917–1918." Spanish Influenza Vertical File. Montana Historical Society Research Center, Helena, MT.

Great Falls Tribune (Great Falls, MT).

Independent Record (Helena, MT).

Montana Code Annotated. 50-2-116. 2017.

Montana Standard (Butte, MT).

Montana State Board of Health Records. Record Series 238. Montana Historical Society Research Center, Helena, MT.

River Press (Fort Benton, MT).

Scobey Sentinel (Scobey, MT).

Silver Bow County. "Report of the Investigation of Sanitary Conditions in Mines, and of the Conditions Under Which the Miners Live in Silver Bow County." 1908–1912. SC89 Montana Historical Society Research Center, Helena, MT.

United States Census Bureau. 1910 United States Census. Silver Bow County, MT.

United States City Directories. 1918. Los Angeles.

Secondary Sources

Barry, John M. *The Great Influenza: The Epic Story of the Deadliest Plague in History*. Rev. ed. New York: Penguin, 2009.

Byerly, Carol. *Fever of War: The Influenza Epidemic in the U.S. Army during World War I*. New York: New York University Press, 2005.

Centers for Disease Control and Prevention. "Avian Influenza A Virus Infections in Humans." Last modified April 18, 2017. www.cdc.gov/flu/avianflu/avian-in-humans.htm.

———. "Disease Burden of Influenza." Last modified May 16, 2017. www.cdc.gov/flu/about/disease/burden.htm.

———. "Highly Pathogenic Asian Avian Influenza A (H5N1) Virus." Last modified October 14, 2015. www.cdc.gov/flu/avianflu/h5n1-virus.htm.

———. "How the Flu Virus Can Change: 'Drift' and 'Shift.'" Last modified September 27, 2017. www.cdc.gov/flu/about/viruses/change.htm.

———. "Influenza A Type Viruses." Last modified April 19, 2017. www.cdc.gov/flu/avianflu/influenza-a-virus-subtypes.htm.

———. "Key Facts about Human Infections with Variant Viruses." Last modified December 21, 2017. www.cdc.gov/flu/swineflu/keyfacts-variant.htm.

———. "Types of *Haemophilus influenzae* Infections." Last modified July 25, 2016. www.cdc.gov/hi-disease/about/types-infection.html.

———. "Types of Influenza Viruses." Last modified September 22, 2017. www.cdc.gov/flu/about/viruses/types.htm.

Coburn, Brian J., Bradley G. Wagner and Sally Blower. "Modeling Influenza Epidemics and Pandemics: Insights into the Future of Swine Flu (H1N1)." *BMC Medicine* 7, no. 3 (2009). bmcmedicine.biomedcentral.com/articles/10.1186/1741-7015-7-30.

Crosby, Alfred W. *America's Forgotten Pandemic: The Influenza of 1918.* 2nd ed. New York: Cambridge University Press, 1989.

Davies, Pete. *The Devil's Flu: The World's Deadliest Influenza Epidemic and the Scientific Hunt for the Virus that Caused It.* New York: Holt Paperbacks, 2000.

Doucleff, Michaeleen. "Anthrax Outbreak in Russia Thought to Be Result of Thawing Permafrost." National Public Radio, August 3, 2016. www. npr.org/sections/goatsandsoda/2016/08/03/488400947/anthrax-outbreak-in-russia-thought-to-be-result-of-thawing-permafrost.

"Dr. Caroline McGill: Mining City Doctor." VF0592. Butte–Silver Bow Public Archives, Butte, MT.

Emmons, David M. *The Butte Irish: Class and Ethnicity in an American Mining Town, 1875–1925.* Urbana: University of Illinois Press, 1990.

Everett, George. "Butte's Far Eastern Influences." 2004. www.butteamerica. com/fareast.htm.

Eyler, John M., PhD. "The State of Science, Microbiology, and Vaccines Circa 1918." *Public Health Reports* 125, suppl. 3 (2010). www.ncbi.nlm.nih. gov/pmc/articles/PMC2862332/.

Garret, Thomas A. "War and Pestilence as Labor Market Shocks: U.S. Manufacturing Wage Growth, 1914–1919." *Economic Inquiry* 47, no. 4 (October 2009): 711–25.

Hoffman, Larry. "The Mining History of Butte and Anaconda." The Mining History Association. Last modified 2011. mininghistoryassociation.org/ ButteHistory.htm.

Howard, Joseph Kinsey. *Montana: High, Wide, and Handsome.* New Haven, CT: Yale University Press, 1943.

"Jeffery Taubenberger." Killer Flu. Public Broadcasting Service. www.pbs. org/wnet/secrets/jeffery-taubenberger/223/.

Katz, Robert S. "Influenza 1918: A Further Study in Mortality." *Bulletin of the History of Medicine* 51, no. 4 (Winter 1977): 617–19.

———. "Influenza 1918: A Study in Mortality." *Bulletin of the History of Medicine* 48, no. 3 (Autumn 1974): 416–22.

Kearney, Pat. *Butte Voices: Mining, Neighborhoods, People.* Butte, MT: Skyhigh Communications, 1998.

Kolata, Gina. *Flu: The Story of the Great Influenza Pandemic of 1918 and the Search for the Virus that Caused It.* New York: Farrar, Straus, and Giroux, 1999.

Luk, Jeffrey, Peter Gross and William W. Thompson. "Observations on Mortality during the 1918 Influenza Pandemic." *Clinical Infectious Diseases* 33, no. 8 (October 15, 2001): 1375–78.

McKenna, Maryn. "Canada's First (and Female) Science Minister Is a Badass." *National Geographic*, November 5, 2015. phenomena. nationalgeographic.com/2015/11/05/canadas-first-and-female-science-minister-is-a-badass/.

"The Medical and Scientific Conceptions of Influenza." virus.stanford.edu/uda/fluscimed.html.

Meyer, Robinson. "The Zombie Diseases of Climate Change." *The Atlantic*, November 6, 2017. www.theatlantic.com/science/archive/2017/11/the-zombie-diseases-of-climate-change/544274/.

Mullen, Pierce C., and Michael L. Nelson. "Montanans and the 'Most Peculiar Disease': The Influenza Epidemic and Public Health, 1918–1999." *Montana: The Magazine of Western History* 37, no. 2 (Spring 1987): 50–61.

Murphy, Mary. *Mining Cultures: Men, Women, and Leisure in Butte, 1914–41.* Urbana: University of Illinois Press, 1997.

"Names and Faces." Mai Wah Society. www.maiwah.org/names.shtml.

Noymer, Andrew, and Michel Garenne. "The 1918 Influenza Epidemic's Effects on Sex Differentials in Mortality in the United States." *Population Development and Review* 26, no. 3 (September 2000): 565–81.

Phillips, Howard, and David Killingray. Introduction to *The Spanish Influenza Pandemic of 1918–1919: New Perspectives.* London: Routledge, 2003.

"Propaganda for Reform." *Journal of the American Medical Association* 71, no. 2 (November 23, 1918).

Punke, Michael. *Fire and Brimstone: The North Butte Mining Disaster of 1917.* New York: Hachette Books, 2007.

Quinn, Tom. *Flu: A Social History of Influenza.* London: New Holland Publishers, 2008.

Rozell, Ned. "Villager's Remains Lead to 1918 Flu Breakthrough." University of Alaska–Fairbanks Geophysical Institute. November 20, 2014. www.gi.alaska.edu/alaska-science-forum/villager-s-remains-lead-1918-flu-breakthrough.

Spinney, Laura. "How the 1918 Flu Pandemic Revolutionized Public Health." *Smithsonian*, September 27, 2017. www.smithsonianmag.com/history/how-1918-flu-pandemic-revolutionized-public-health-180965025/.

Stanford News Service. "Wayne S. Vucinich, Father of East European Studies, Dead at 91." Stanford University Palo Alto, CA), April 28, 2005. news.stanford.edu/pr/2005/pr-obitwayne-042705.html.

Steele, Volney. "The Flu Epidemic of 1918 on the Montana Frontier." *Journal of the West* 42 no. 4 (Fall 2003): 81–90.

Taubenberger, Jeffery K., and David M. Morens. "1918 Influenza: The Mother of all Pandemics." *Emerging Infectious Diseases* 12, no. 1 (January 2006). www.ncbi.nlm.nih.gov/pmc/articles/PMC3291398/.

Taylor, Michael. "Wayne Vucinich—Stanford History Professor." *SF Gate*, May 1, 2005. www.sfgate.com/bayarea/article/Wayne-Vucinich-Stanford-history-professor-2676537.php.

Toole, K. Ross. *Twentieth-Century Montana: A State of Extremes.* Norman: University of Oklahoma Press, 1972.

Visnes Mine Museum. visitkarmoy.no/en/vigsnes-grubemuseum.

Waldrup, Hal. "Huie Pock: Pioneer Chinese Doctor." Montana Writers' Workshop. VF1061. Butte–Silver Bow Public Archives, Butte, MT.

Walters, John H., MD. "Influenza 1918: The Contemporary Perspective." *Bulletin of the New York Academy of Medicine* 54, no. 9 (October 1978): 855–64.

Writers' Project of Montana. *Copper Camp: Stories of the World's Greatest Mining Town, Butte, Montana.* Helena, MT: Riverbend Publishing, 1943.

Yong, Ed. "The Deadly Panic-Neglect Cycle in Pandemic Funding." *The Atlantic*, October 24, 2017. www.theatlantic.com/science/archive/2017/10/panic-neglect-pandemic-funding/543696/.

ABOUT THE AUTHOR

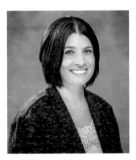

Janelle M. Olberding is an independent historian, writer, avid reader, part-time educator, and lifelong learner. She holds a vested interest in public health and worked in the field of public health preparedness and communicable disease prevention for six years. She currently works in higher education and lives in Glendive, Montana, with her husband and daughter.

Visit us at
www.historypress.com